PR
OBSTETR
Analysis a... Management

Problems in Anaesthesia

Titles in the series

Problems in Anaesthesia: Analysis and Management
S. Feldman, W. Harrop-Griffiths and N. Hirsch

Life-Threatening Problems in the Emergency Room
A. Sutcliffe

Problems in Obstetric Anaesthesia: Analysis and Management
A. Rubin and M. Wood

Titles in preparation

Problems in Intensive Care: Analysis and Management
N. Soni and W. Harrop-Griffiths

PROBLEMS IN OBSTETRIC ANAESTHESIA
Analysis and Management

Problems in Anaesthesia

Anthony P. Rubin
MB, BChir, MRCS, LRCP, FFARCS, DA

*Consultant Anaesthetist, Charing Cross Hospital,
London, UK*

and

Matthew L. B. Wood
MB, ChB, MRCP, FFARCS

*Anaesthetic Senior Registrar, St George's Hospital,
London, UK; Visiting Associate Professor, Department of
Anesthesiology, Duke University Medical Center, Durham,
North Carolina, USA*

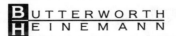

BUTTERWORTH
HEINEMANN

Butterworth-Heinemann Ltd
Linacre House, Jordan Hill, Oxford OX2 8DP

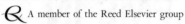 A member of the Reed Elsevier group

OXFORD LONDON BOSTON
MUNICH NEW DELHI SINGAPORE SYDNEY
TOKYO TORONTO WELLINGTON

First published 1993

British Library Cataloguing in Publication Data
Rubin, Anthony P.
  Problems in Obstetric Anaesthesia:
  Analysis and Management. – (Problems in
  Anaesthesia Series)
  I. Title II. Wood, Matthew L. B.
  III. Series
  617.9

ISBN 0 7506 0710 6

Library of Congress Cataloguing in Publication Data
Rubin, Anthony P.
  Problems in obstetric anaesthesia: analysis and management/
  Anthony P. Rubin, Matthew L.B. Wood.
  p. cm. —(Problems in anaesthesia)
  ISBN 0 7506 0710 6
  1. Anesthesia in obstetrics—Complications. I. Wood, Matthew L.
  B. II. Title. III. Series.
  [DNLM: 1. Anesthesia, Obstetrical. 2. Pregnancy Complications.
  WO 450 R896p 1993]
  RG732.R83 1993
  617.9'682—dc20
  DNLM/DLC
  for Library of Congress   92-48412
                                                              CIP

Set 10 on 11 point Times by
P&R Typesetters Ltd, Salisbury, Wilts

Printed in Great Britain at the University Press, Cambridge

Contents

Foreword   vii

Preface   ix

Section one. Coexisting disease and pregnancy   **1**
Introduction   3
Cardiovascular disease   3
Asthma   8
Neurological disease   13
Diabetes   16
Obesity   20
Anaemia   23
Sickle cell disease   25

Section two. Regional anaesthesia in obstetrics   **29**
Introduction   31
Anatomy and physiology   31
Extradural analgesia for labour and operative delivery   33
Inadequate extradural analgesia   35
Extensive block   38
Bloody tap   40
Toxic reaction to local anaesthetics   41
Urinary retention   45
Dural puncture headache   46
Shivering   48
Broken extradural catheter   49
Prolonged neurological deficit   49
Extradural haematoma and abscess   51

Section three. Emergencies   **53**
Cardiac arrest   55
Haemorrhage   59
Haemostatic failure   64
Embolism   67
Cyanosis   74
Convulsions   76

Contents

Anaphylactoid reactions 79
Difficult intubation 83
Aspiration of gastric contents 89
Post-operative respiratory difficulties 92
Resuscitation of the neonate 98

Section four. Miscellaneous **103**
Pre-eclampsia 105
Anaesthesia during pregnancy 109
Awareness 111
Abnormal labour and delivery 114

Appendix I. Physiological changes of pregnancy **121**

Appendix II. Drugs used in obstetric anaesthetic practice **125**

Index **131**

Foreword

Education in medicine and the long training of a specialist anaesthetist give a sound background of scientific and clinical information allowing assessment of the possible risks of any proposed treatment against the potential benefit to the patient. This risk-benefit analysis is fundamental to all doctors presented with a medical problem.

Nowhere is this concept of greater importance than in the treatment of problems in obstetric anaesthesia where rapid decisions which may be a matter of life or death or result in a tragically damaged baby are essential. Because much obstetric care is provided by non-physician personnel many of the regimes of treatment are by protocol or mandated algorithms. Whilst this may be a framework to allow differing specialities to understand each other's role, they should not restrict the specialist anaesthetist's ability to select the most appropriate therapy for a patient in a particular set of circumstances. However, in order to decide upon the most suitable treatment it is necessary first to diagnose the condition accurately and to consider the problem it poses to the patient's physiology and the pharmacological implications it may have on any drugs administered.

In the *Problems in Anaesthesia* series this approach has been used to explain the objectives of the treatment recommended. In this book, common obstetric problems are analysed and defined and the pathological and physiological consequences analysed. Any pharmacological implications of the process are presented. This leads to a rational presentation of therapeutic options. In this way the book points the way to logical decision making in obstetrics.

A small book of this sort is not meant to be a definitive treatise on obstetric anaesthesia, but rather a companion to the anaesthetist in training, a revision source for those who have not recently been involved in anaesthetising women in labour and a source of information for those about to start obstetric anaesthesia.

Professor S. Feldman

Preface

Providing anaesthetic cover for the labour ward is one of the responsibilities that falls to the trainee anaesthetist as they progress in a career in anaesthesia. The prospect of such responsibilities is understandably daunting and the first months working on the obstetric unit are often stressful for anaesthetists who are experienced in applying their skills to provide anaesthesia for elective and emergency general, urological and gynaecological surgery but whose exposure to the problems peculiar to obstetric anaesthesia are limited.

The purpose of this book is to provide anaesthetists at such a stage in their training with an indication of the sorts of situations that they may reasonably expect to see in everyday obstetric practice and a guide to the management of such situations. It is hoped that the format of the book will allow it to be kept in a pocket and easily referred to at short notice when a situation is encountered for the first time and also as an aide memoir to those more experienced anaesthetists.

We have attempted to present each subject in a consistent format: a definition of the problem; how to make the diagnosis; its possible causes where appropriate; the physiological significance of the condition to the mother and fetus; how to assess the state of the mother; and how to manage the problem in terms of providing analgesia during labour and anaesthesia for operative delivery.

Some points that should be remembered when confronted by any situation in obstetric anaesthesia:

1. The pregnant woman comprises two people; the mother and the fetus. Changes seen in the mother such as hypotension will have adverse effects on the fetus if not treated promptly.
2. The maintenance of adequate oxygenation and placental perfusion are the goals of treatment of the sick pregnant woman.

3. All pregnant women after the fist trimester are at risk of aspiration of gastric contents during general anaesthesia and for this reason regional anaesthesia should be used wherever possible.
4. Aorto-caval compression must be anticipated and treated in all pregnant women by lateral displacement of the uterus either manually or by positioning the mother in the wedged or lateral position.
5. Always summon senior anaesthetic assistance when significant problems are anticipated, or if not anticipated then very soon after difficulties arise.

Coexisting disease and pregnancy

Introduction

Mothers may have a coexisting illness which may have implications for those involved in the care of the mother and fetus.

The purpose of this section is to provide the trainee anaesthetist with a guide to the types of conditions that may present in a general obstetric unit; advice on how to assess their severity to allow meaningful communication between trainee and senior; and how to manage these conditions definitively or while awaiting the arrival of senior help.

Cardiovascular disease

The incidence of cardiac disease in pregnancy is low (0.4–2%) but it is a significant non-obstetric cause of maternal mortality. The relative incidence of congenital heart disease has increased because of more patients survive to childbearing age following corrective surgery. The types of problems encountered include:

- Valvular lesions
  —aortic stenosis/insufficiency
  —mitral stenosis/insufficiency
  —mixed lesions
- Prosthetic heart valves
- Left-to-right shunts
  —ventricular septal defect (VSD)
  —atrial septal defect (ASD)
  —patent ductus arteriosus (PDA)
- Right-to-left shunts
  —Tetralogy of Fallot
  —Eisenmenger's syndrome
  —pulmonary hypertension

- Peripartum cardiomyopathy
- Coronary artery disease
- Arrhythmias

Physiological significance. There is an increase in blood volume and cardiac output in pregnancy (Appendix I) which may cause decompensation of an already compromised cardiovascular system especially during the demanding peripartum period.

The risks of maternal morbidity, maternal mortality and perinatal mortality are determined by three factors:

1. The underlying lesion
2. The functional compromise due to the lesion
3. Associated pregnancy-related complications e.g. pre-eclampsia, haemorrhage and infection

Assessment of the mother

History. Symptoms of heart disease in the non-obstetric patient, dyspnoea, palpitations, tiredness, weight gain and oedema are common complaints in pregnancy, so a history of antenatal symptoms and any changes since the onset of pregnancy should be elicited. Syncope is unusual in normal pregnancy unless there is aortocaval compression and should be considered a significant symptom. On the basis of this history mothers can be graded according to the New York Heart Association (NYHA) functional impairment classification (see Table 1.1).

Conditions in which pregnancy is well tolerated (less than 1% mortality) are:

Septal defects
Patent ductus arteriosus
Corrected Tetralogy of Fallot
Corrected coarctation of the aorta
Pre-existing arrhythmias
NYHA classes I and II

Table 1.1 NYHA functional classification of cardiac disease

Class I	No functional limitation of activity
	No symptoms of decompensation with activity
Class II	Mild amount of functional limitation
	Asymptomatic at rest
	Ordinary physical activity causes symptoms
Class III	Limitation of most physical activity
	Asymptomatic at rest
	Minimal physical activity causes symptoms
Class IV	Severe limitation of physical activity
	May be symptomatic at rest
	Any physical activity causes cardiac symptoms

Examination. Signs of the suspected lesion and cardiac failure should be elicited and their presence confirmed by relevant investigation.

The signs of cardiac failure are:

- Tachycardia
- Tachypnoea
- Triple rhythm
- Distended neck veins
- Oedema

The patient's records should be checked for details of pre-existing cardiac problems and results of previous investigations compared with any performed during this confinement.

Investigations. Non-invasive investigations which should be considered include:

- ECG
- Chest X-ray
- Echocardiography
  —diagnosis of lesion
  —assessment of ventricular function

- 24-hour ECG
  —diagnosis of causes of syncope and palpitations
- Pulse oximetry
  —assessment of shunting
- Serial vital capacity
  —decreases with pulmonary oedema

Management during labour and delivery. Management of the parturient with cardiovascular disease requires the co-ordinated involvement of an experienced obstetrician, cardiologist and anaesthetist. Patients with NYHA classification III and IV require invasive monitoring (pulmonary artery catheter) during labour and delivery.

Certain lesions predispose the mother to bacterial endocarditis. Antibiotic prophylaxis is recommended in all patients with prosthetic heart valves and congenital malformations except isolated secundum atrial septal defect (ASD).

Recommended regimen
No allergy to penicillin: Ampicillin 2 g plus Gentamicin 120 mg i.v./i.m. at the start of labour or induction and repeated once 8 hours later.

Allergic to penicillin: Vancomycin 1 g i.v. (given over 60 minutes in 100 ml 5% dextrose) plus Gentamicin 120 mg i.v./i.m. at the start of labour or induction and repeated once 8 hours later.

Analgesia during labour. Extradural analgesia is the technique of choice in those patients with cardiac disease without contraindications which include anticoagulation, hypovolaemia or fixed cardiac output states (e.g. stenotic valve disease, pericarditis). By providing good analgesia by afferent block, extradural analgesia reduces both the stress response (increased catecholamine, steroid and ADH release) and the demands made on the heart during labour and delivery.

Slow incremental administration of local anaesthetic during extradural block and judicious use of intravenous fluids and vasoconstrictors minimizes any hypotension which is undesirable in the cardiac patient.

When extradural analgesia is contraindicated Entonox inhalation or parenteral opiates are suitable alternatives.

Operative procedures. Extradural block with slow incremental administration of local anaesthetic is the technique of choice in the absence of contraindications, for the reasons given above. The use of an indwelling extradural catheter allows optimal analgesia and attenuates the stress of a painful post operative period. The rapid, profound sympathetic block and hypotension associated with subarachnoid block makes the use of the technique undesirable.

Where general anaesthesia is required because of emergency or contraindication to use of extradural block consideration should be given to the needs and implications of a cardiac anaesthetic. Tracheal intubation is required in the obstetric patient but is associated with a significant pressor response and arrhythmias. To attenuate this response several measures may be taken including the use of moderate dose opiates (alfentanil 5 µg/kg) for induction, beta-blockade (esmolol 500 µg bolus) or intravenous lignocaine (1–2 mg/kg) given prior to intubation. High-dose opiates may cause respiratory depression of the neonate. Beta-blockade and lignocaine are not well tolerated by patients with severe myocardial compromise.

The recommended technique is

- Pre-oxygenation
- Cricoid pressure
- Rapid sequence i.v. induction with thiopentone (3–5 mg/kg) and suxamethonium (1–1.5 mg/kg); alfentanil (5 µg/kg) bolus prior to intubation; nitrous oxide/oxygen and enflurane 0.6–1% inspired concentration and vecuronium (0.1 mg/kg). The use of air rather than nitrous oxide should be considered in the unstable patient because of the myocardial depressant effect of nitrous oxide.

Reversal with neostigmine (50 µg/kg) and glycopyrollate (10 µg/kg) rather than atropine should be used to avoid tachycardia.

The mother should be transferred to a High Dependency Unit post-operatively for continued cardiovascular monitoring and support if necessary.

Asthma

Although pregnancy imposes increased demands on the respiratory system in terms of increased oxygen consumption and carbon dioxide elimination, significant decompensation due to respiratory disease is rare.

Asthma is the commonest respiratory problem occurring in approximately 1% of pregnancies.

The obstetric anaesthetist may be involved in the management of a mother suffering a serious asthmatic attack at any stage in the antenatal period. They should be able to initiate and manage the first line treatment and be able to assess the need for more intensive therapy including ventilatory support. Although acute attacks are rare in the final month of pregnancy or during labour the advice of the anaesthetist should be sought for the management of analgesia during labour.

Definition. Asthma is a condition characterized by recurrent dyspnoea secondary to limitation of bronchial airflow as a result of bronchospasm, bronchial oedema and mucus plugs, produced in response to a variety of stimuli.

Physiological significance. The effect of pregnancy on the severity of asthma is variable but in the majority of patients it either improves or is unchanged. It remains a source of morbidity and mortality which can only be minimized if managed correctly and with care.

For the fetus severe maternal hypoxia (pO_2<8 kPa) can be fatal.

Assessment of the mother

History. Details obtained should include:
- Severity of dyspnoea
- Presence, severity and frequency of any wheeze
- Existence of cough and whether it is productive
- Fever
- Duration of symptoms
- Precipitating factors of this and previous attacks
- Previous admissions especially to intensive therapy unit
- Drug therapy
  —bronchodilators
  —high-dose steroids
  —missed doses of regular medication
- Questioning about the coexistence of other cardiorespiratory disease

'High risk' patients are those with an increased frequency of attacks, previous admission especially if mechanical ventilation was required, a long delay in presenting for treatment and if taking high-dose steroid therapy.

Examination
- General appearance: use of accessory respiratory muscles, distress and exhaustion, level of consciousness and state of hydration
- Temperature
- Respiratory rate
- Dyspnoea
- Wheezing
- Heart rate
- Presence and degree of pulsus paradoxus – a fall in systolic pressure during inspiration >20 mmHg is considered significant

Investigations. Investigation of the patient should include the performance of:

- Full blood count
- Serum urea and electrolytes
- Arterial blood gases (ABG)
- Spirometry
- Peak expiratory flow rate (PEFR)
- Microscopy and culture of sputum
- Chest X-ray to exclude bronchopneumonia and pneumothorax

Indicators of a severe asthma attack include:

- A heart rate >120 beats per minute
- Pulsus paradoxus >20 mmHg
- Moderate to severe dyspnoea and wheeze
- A respiratory rate >30 breaths per minute
- The use of accessory muscles of respiration
- Peak expiratory flow rate (PEFR) <120 litres per minute

Management

Acute asthmatic attack. Treatment in the pregnant patient is no different to that of the non-pregnant asthmatic and all the therapies used are safe in pregnancy.

The prevention and treatment of hypoxia are vital in pregnancy because of the danger to the fetus.

The components of therapy should comprise:

1. Humidified oxygen
   —inspired oxygen concentration increased as required to maintain $PaO_2 > 10$ kPa
2. i.v. fluids
   —replacement and maintenance (4 ml/kg/hr dextrose saline solution)

3. Beta-agonists
   —nebulized salbutamol 2.5–5 mg in 2 ml saline 6 hourly, the initial dose may be repeated after 30 minutes as necessary, up to three doses at the onset of therapy
4. Aminophylline
   —loading dose 6 mg/kg in 100 ml dextrose i.v. over 30 minutes, maintenance dose 0.5–0.7 mg/kg per hour to maintain serum levels in the therapeutic range 10–20 μg per ml
5. Glucocorticoids
   —hydrocortisone 100–200 mg i.v. 6 hourly
6. Antibiotics
   —where bronchopneumonia is suspected
   ampicillin 500 mg i.v. 6 hourly
   or
   erythromycin 500 mg i.v. 6 hourly
7. Regular assessment
   —hourly PEFR and ABGs during early period of treatment

In the pregnant patient arterial blood gases are the most useful indicator of the severity of the attack and must be interpreted with reference to the normal arterial blood gases seen in pregnancy (Appendix I) which show a compensated respiratory alkalosis. Patients with pH<7.35 and pCO_2>5 kPa should be considered as candidates for intensive care and if any further deterioration of arterial blood gases with increasing fatigue occur, mechanical ventilation should be instituted.

Labour and delivery. The patient's regular bronchodilator therapy should be continued throughout the peripartum period.

Syntocinon can be safely used for augmentation of labour but prostaglandins should be avoided because of the risk of precipitation of bronchospasm.

Analgesia for labour. Extradural analgesia provided by local anaesthetics is the technique of choice in the absence of any contraindications (q.v.) because of the reduced demands on the respiratory system produced by effective analgesia.

Where regional analgesia is contraindicated and Entonox is inadequate parenteral pethidine (0.5–1 mg/kg i.v./i.m.) is relatively safe in the absence of wheeze or respiratory compromise.

Operative delivery. Elective caesarean section should not be performed on a patient whose bronchospasm is not optimally controlled.

Regional anaesthesia. In the absence of any contraindication or requirement for immediate delivery, extradural block is the technique of choice for instrumental delivery or caesarean section.

If the parturient experiences pain during surgery because of an insufficiently dense block small intravenous boluses (25–50 µg) of fentanyl may be used to supplement the block.

Fentanyl (50–100 µg) may be safely given, into the epidural space, during or at the end of surgery to provide 3–4 hours of post operative analgesia. The asthmatic patient may be uncomfortable in the supine position for extended periods and should have a slight head-up tilt or extra pillow props.

General anaesthesia. If general anaesthesia is required a rapid sequence induction and balanced anaesthetic technique should be used. The drugs of choice are:

- Etomidate 0.2–0.3 mg/kg or ketamine 1–2 mg/kg
- Suxamethonium 1–1.5 mg/kg
- Vecuronium 0.1 mg/kg
- Isoflurane (0.5–0.75%) or enflurane (0.6–1%)
    —halothane is not recommended in conjunction with B-agonist therapy because of its dysrhythmic potential
- Pethidine 1–1.5 mg/kg or fentanyl 2–5 µg/kg as analgesia after delivery of fetus
- Ventilation should be provided at a slow rate; with a large tidal volume and a low I:E ratio
- Post-operative analgesia can be safely achieved with either pethidine 0.5–1 mg/kg i.m. 3 hourly or pethidine 0.1–0.3 mg/kg/hour by i.v. infusion

Neurological disease

Neurological disorders may be acute e.g. cerebral tumour, or chronic e.g. paraplegia. Furthermore, patients may suffer acute exacerbations of a chronic disorder such as multiple sclerosis.

Few conditions have an adverse effect on the course of pregnancy, but pregnancy may have a variable effect on the relapse rate or exacerbation of an underlying neurological or neuromuscular disorder.

A comprehensive discussion of all neurological conditions is beyond the scope of this book. The management of three of the more frequently seen conditions are described to illustrate the principles of management of the parturient with a coexisting neuromuscular disease.

Physiological significance. Neurological and neuromuscular disease may interfere with respiratory function and control of upper airway protective reflexes. The myocardium may be involved in some neuromuscular disorders such as myotonic dystrophy leading to dysrhythmias and heart failure.

Patients with long-standing neurological disease may suffer the complications of immobility such as contractures, pressure sores or renal stones.

Assessment of mother. When making a pre-anaesthetic assessment of a mother the anaesthetist must attempt to quantify and record the degree of:
- Motor and sensory deficit
- Respiratory function
  —gag reflex
  —vitalography – vital capacity
- Cardiovascular function
  —ECG
  —echocardiography
- Miscellaneous
  —drug therapy
  —pressure areas
  —renal function

Management

Paraplegia. If the level of sensory loss is higher than T10 then labour and delivery will be painless.

The aim of management is to provide adequate analgesia where necessary and prevent the autonomic disturbance which occurs in response to distension of the uterus or bladder and the mass motor reflex that occurs below the level of the cord lesion.

Features of the autonomic disturbance include:

- Malignant rise in blood pressure
- Bradycardia
- Sweating

Extradural and subarachnoid block prevent these reflexes and are the techniques of choice for both analgesia in labour and for operative delivery. Hypotension can be effectively and safely treated with ephedrine (10–15 mg i.v.).

If general anaesthesia is required the use of suxamethonium within 12 months of the injury may cause hyperkalaemia.

Multiple sclerosis. The course of pregnancy and labour is unaffected by multiple sclerosis and pregnancy does not affect the relapse rate, but there is an increased rate of relapse in the postpartum period.

Stress and pyrexia are factors known to cause relapse.

Extradural block provides optimal analgesia for labour and delivery and reduces stress and spasticity. Although the overall rate of relapse rate is no higher after extradural block the lowest possible concentration of local anaesthetic is recommended since relapse rate may be directly related to anaesthetic concentration. For this reason subarachnoid block is not advised. The addition of 50–100 µg fentanyl to the local anaesthetic may allow lower concentrations to be effective.

For operative delivery extradural block is not contra-indicated. General anaesthesia does not have any adverse effects on multiple sclerosis but attention should be paid to temperature regulation and post-operative respiratory function and protection of the airway if bulbar or pseudobulbar palsy is present.

This information should be given to the parturient when obtaining consent prior to performing an extradural block.

Myasthenia gravis. Pregnancy has no consistent effect on the course of myasthenia gravis. Up to 20% of neonates born to mothers with myasthenia may develop symptoms of the disease up to 4 days after delivery.

Parenteral anticholinesterase therapy should be continued; vital capacity measured and bulbar weakness (gag reflex) assessed throughout labour.

Drugs known to exacerbate myasthenia which may be seen in use during labour and which are contraindicated in the myasthenic parturient include:

gentamicin	antibiotic
propranolol	antihypertensive
ritodrine	tocolytic
terbutaline	bronchodilator

Extradural block may be used as analgesia for labour and delivery. If the local anaesthetic is given slowly, to allow frequent assessment of motor block, it provides good quality analgesia and avoids the risk of respiratory depression of opiate analgesics, to which the myasthenic is very sensitive.

Regional anaesthesia is also recommended for operative delivery providing respiratory and bulbar muscle function is adequate to allow spontaneous respiration and protection of the airway.

An indwelling extradural catheter can be used to provide post-operative analgesia.

If general anaesthesia is indicated a rapid sequence technique should be performed using thiopentone and suxamethonium (to which the myasthenic may be resistant).

The myasthenic is exquisitely sensitive to non-depolarizing muscle relaxants. Small doses should be used (atracurium 0.02–0.04 mg/kg) and the effect monitored with a peripheral nerve stimulator. The lowest doses of depressant drugs, e.g. volatile agents and opiate analgesics, that provide adequate anaesthesia and analgesia should be used.

Reversal of muscle block with i.v. neostigmine should be given in increments (0.5 mg i.v.) and the patient extubated when fully awake; when a return of twitch to pre-operative height and the patient able to generate a vital capacity >30 ml/kg.

Post-operatively patients should be given oxygen for 24 hours after delivery; recommenced on anticholinesterase therapy and vital capacity and other muscle function monitored regularly until anticholinesterase requirements have stabilized.

Post-operative analgesia should be with small doses of intravenous opiates or by means of continuous extradural block if there are no contraindications to insertion of an extradural catheter.

Diabetes

Definition.   Pregnancy induced diabetes is defined as carbohydrate intolerance of variable severity that has its onset or diagnosis during pregnancy.

Diabetes may antedate pregnancy and may be managed by dietary control, oral hypoglycaemic drugs or by insulin therapy.

Physiological significance.   Diabetes is characterized by damage to several organs leading to:

- Coronary artery disease
- Cerebrovascular disease
- Nephropathy
- Retinopathy
- Neuropathy
  —autonomic
  —peripheral

The pathogenesis of such damage is large and small vessel disease.

Mother. The pregnant diabetic is likely to suffer a deterioration of her glycaemic control during pregnancy and is at an increased risk of pregnancy induced hypertension. She is more likely to have a large baby leading to prolonged labour, birth trauma and fetal asphyxia.

Fetus. The fetus of the diabetic parturient is at risk of congenital malformation, prematurity, hypoxia, acidosis and sudden late intrauterine death.

For these reasons the incidence of caesarean section is as high as 50%.

Assessment of the mother

History. From the history the following should be established

- The duration of diabetes
- Glycaemic therapy
  —day-to-day
  —following previous anaesthesia
- The quality of glycaemic control
  —hyperglycaemia
  —hypoglycaemic episodes
  —admissions with ketoacidosis
- Complications of diabetes
  —cardiovascular disease
  —hypertension
  —renal disease
  —neuropathy/retinopathy
  —infections
- Drug history
  —oral hypoglycaemic and insulin therapy: type, names and doses
  —antihypertensives

Examination. During the examination the clinician should look for signs of organ damage due to diabetes:

- Cardiovascular – blood pressure including lying and standing to assess postural hypotension
- Neurological – the presence of sensory or motor neuropathy
- Airway – assessment of jaw opening ('stiff joint syndrome')
- Skin – inspection of the lumbar spine for infected skin lesions

Investigations. The results of the following investigation should be known:

- Full blood count
- Glycosylated haemoglobin – <8% suggests good glycaemic control
- Urea, creatinine and electrolytes
- Fasting blood glucose
- ECG
- Urinalysis with special attention to ketonuria

Management. It is usual to plan delivery at 38–40 weeks to avoid the risk of late intrauterine death. Delivery is by caesarean section if the fetus is suspected of being large or is compromised.

Intrapartum period

Blood glucose control. Good control is vital and the optimal blood glucose is 4.5–5.5 mmol/l. Hypoglycaemia is potentially harmful to the mother and also inhibits uterine action. Hyperglycaemia carries the risk of neonatal hypoglycaemia.

Oral hypoglycaemics should be stopped 48 hours prior to delivery.

Intrapartum dextrose/insulin regimen:

- 5% Dextrose 1000 ml i.v. 8 hourly
- Check BM stix 2 hourly – if BM<3.5 mmol/l increase rate of dextrose infusion and if necessary change to 10% dextrose
- Insulin infusion as per sliding scale:

  For example

BM stix (mmol/l)	Insulin (ml/hr) (50 u soluble insulin in 50 ml N-saline)
0–5	0.5
5–10	2
10–15	4
15–20	8
>20	Check with a formal laboratory specimen rather than a BM stix

- Check the serum potassium 4 hourly – if K$^+$<3.5 mmol/l add 20 mmol of KCl to each litre of dextrose

Postpartum period.
- Pre-pregnancy diabetes – return to antenatal hypoglycaemic regimen
- Gestational diabetes – stop insulin therapy immediately after delivery.

Analgesia for labour. Catecholamines and glucocorticoids released in response to the pain of labour increase resistance to insulin. Continuous lumbar extradural analgesia attenuates this response and is the method of choice for pain relief in labour. Extradural analgesia is less likely than opiates to cause nausea which may delay the resumption of oral intake and therefore usual glycaemic therapy in the postpartum period.

Operative delivery. Subarachnoid or extradural blocks are advised to avoid the metabolic and dietary disturbance associated with general anaesthesia.

Accurate control of blood pressure is particularly important because the fetus is at increased risk of hypoxia and acidosis.

Non-glucose containing crystalloid solutions should be used to avoid hypotension and should be administered via a separate port to that of the maintenance dextrose solution.

If general anaesthesia is necessary anaesthetists should remember the possibility of 'stiff-joint syndrome' in the young insulin dependent diabetic, causing possible difficulty with tracheal intubation.

Obesity

Approximately 6% of pregnant patients are obese. Obesity in pregnancy provides physiological challenges to the mother and technical problems to the anaesthetist, obstetrician and other staff working on the labour ward.

Definition.   A patient is defined as obese when they weigh 20% more than their ideal body weight (height in centimetres minus 105 = weight in kg), and morbidly obese when weighing 70% more.

Physiological significance

Mother.   Obesity significantly increases morbidity and mortality of the non-pregnant patient from several conditions including: hypertension, diabetes, cerebrovascular, thromboembolic and liver disease.

The obese parturient is at further increased risk of diseases associated with pregnancy: pre-eclampsia, gestational diabetes, and deep vein thrombosis and pulmonary embolism. cerebrovascular disease, as well as sudden death in the supine position.

Fetus.   The fetus is more likely to become distressed and there is an increased perinatal mortality rate if the mother suffers any antenatal medical complications.

Umbilical cord prolapse, shoulder dystocia and fetal distress are more common, making emergency caesarean section more likely. Blood loss during caesarean section is likely to exceed 1000 ml.

Assessment

History.   The mother should be asked about:

- The duration of obesity
- Previous anaesthetics and whether there were any problems
- Associated medical conditions
- Recent significant weight changes

Examination.   The following should be included in the examination:

- Observation to make a general assessment of the degree of obesity
- Measurement of height and weight which is often not possible
- Calculation of ideal body weight
- Airway assessment
- Presence and ease of venous access
- The lumbar spine
- Evidence of associated medical conditions

Investigations.   Minimum investigations should comprise:

- Full blood count
- Plasma urea, electrolytes and glucose
- ECG
- Arterial blood gases

The implications for the management of the obese parturient are legion and affect all members of the obstetric team. It is important that the anaesthetist assembles adequate numbers of personnel to help during the movement of the patient, induction of anaesthesia and post-operatively.

The following should be considered when managing the obese parturient:

- Mechanical problems
  —moving the patient
  —size of operating table
  —the need for arm supports and a suitably sized wedge
- Cardiovascular problems
  —difficulty monitoring blood pressure – a large cuff is required
  —higher incidence of aortocaval compression
  —greater amount of blood loss
  —increased incidence of thromboembolism
- Respiratory problems
  —possible difficulty in airway management
  —rapid desaturation during apnoea
  —peri-operative hypoxaemia
  —increased likelihood of post-operative respiratory difficulties
- Gastrointestinal
  —an increased risk of reflux because of delayed gastric emptying; increased gastric volume and decreased gastric pH
- Technical problems
  —difficulty achieving good venous access
  —trouble identifying landmarks and depth of the extradural or subarachnoid space

Analgesia for labour. Despite potential technical difficulties continuous lumbar extradural analgesia is recommended. The assistance of a senior anaesthetist should be sought if technically difficult. Long Tuohy needles are rarely required.

Operative delivery. Lumbar extradural block via an indwelling extradural catheter is the technique of choice because it allows optimal post-operative analgesia.

If general anaesthesia is required the technique is the same as for the non-obese parturient but the anaesthetist should remember:

1. To give antacid therapy
2. To pre-oxygenate for 5 minutes
3. That more than 500 mg of thiopentone is rarely required
4. To give the normal dose of suxamethonium, 1.5 mg/kg
5. The need for equipment for difficult intubation
   —gum elastic bougie
   —long blade for the laryngoscope

It is recommended that the patient should be transferred to a high dependency area in the immediate post-operative period for management of post-operative analgesia, oxygen therapy and monitoring of respiratory function for 24 hours.

Anaemia

Definition. Anaemia is a concentration of haemoglobin below that expected in someone of a given age, sex and racial origin.

Haemoglobin concentration may fall due to: an increased loss of erythrocytes, inadequate erythropoiesis, increased erythrocyte destruction or haemodilution.

In pregnancy a 'physiological anaemia' occurs because of a disparity in the increase in plasma volume and red cell mass causing haemodilution. Despite this, haemoglobin should not fall to less than 12 g% in the final trimester, provided iron supplements are taken throughout pregnancy.

Physiological significance. Both mother and fetus require an adequate supply of oxygen to maintain organ function. The total oxygen available to the tissues, or 'oxygen flux' is a function of the oxygen carrying capacity of the blood and the cardiac output (see below)

$$\frac{\text{Oxygen flux}}{(\text{ml/min})} = \frac{CO \times SaO_2 \times Hb \times 1.39}{10}$$

CO = cardiac output (l/min)
SaO_2 = arterial oxygen saturation of haemoglobin (%)
Hb = haemoglobin concentration (g/dl)
1.39 = oxygen capacity of haemoglobin (ml/g)

Any fall in oxygen carrying capacity due to anaemia should be compensated for by an increase in cardiac output.

In pregnancy there is a 40% increase in cardiac output and the reduction of haematocrit (35%) improves the flow characteristics of blood through vascular beds thus maintaining carriage of oxygen. However any pre-existing cardiovascular disease or anaemia in the parturient may prevent these compensatory changes. The extra oxygen demands of pregnancy (20%) and either labour or operative delivery may lead to cardiovascular decompensation unless haemoglobin concentration is increased with a blood transfusion.

Management. The anaesthetist may be presented with a mother presenting for elective caesarean section with a low haemoglobin, and should decide whether the case should be postponed or what haemoglobin is acceptable for anaesthesia.

For the previously well mother with anaemia who is asymptomatic and undergoing her first caesarean section, pre-operative transfusion is unnecessary and any transfusion can be postponed until a post-operative haemoglobin concentration has been measured. Even then if the mother feels well, transfusion may be avoided and haematinic therapy used as an alternative.

Treatment of anaemia by means of either haematinic therapy or transfusion in patients with renal failure or thalassaemia may be inappropriate because of the dangers of iron overload and suppression of erythropoiesis.

In the case of the mother with pre-existing cardiac or respiratory disease careful pre-operative and early intra-operative transfusion is indicated, with attention paid to the risk of fluid overload in those mothers with cardiac failure.

When emergency surgery is necessary pre-operative haemo-globin concentration may not be available as a guide to trans-fusion requirements and circumstances do not allow for delay, but reference to haemoglobin assays performed during last trimester antenatal clinic visits provide a useful estimate pro-viding there has been no blood loss since the visit to the clinic.

During anaesthesia the anaesthetist should maintain circu-lating blood volume, cardiac output and FiO_2 to maximize oxygen flux.

Sickle cell disease

Definition. Sickle cell disease is a syndrome caused by the distortion of red blood cells by the polymerization of abnormal haemoglobin molecules under conditions of low pH, stasis and hypoxia.

There are several inherited haemoglobinopathies that can be distinguished by electrophoresis. The commonest is true sickle cell anaemia (homozygous, HbSS), others include sickle cell trait (heterozygous, HbSA), haemoglobin C disease (HbSC) and sickle thalassaemia (HbS-β Thal).

The clinical features are characterized by episodic 'crises' which may be one or all of the following:

- *vaso-occlusive* causing infarction, pain and organ damage
- *haemolytic* leading to jaundice and abdominal pain
- *aplastic* – acute bone marrow depression resulting in anaemia

Significance. Pregnancy and labour have an adverse effect on the sickling process. The *mother* has an increased morbidity and mortality. She is more likely to suffer from pre-eclampsia, respiratory and urinary tract infections, anaemia and thrombosis.

Perinatal mortality is four times the normal and the *fetus* is more likely to be born prematurely, be small for dates and suffer fetal distress.

For these reasons the obstetric anaesthetist is likely to be involved in the peripartum management of these patients who are considered to have high-risk pregnancies.

Assessment

History. From the history the following should be established:

- The occurrence and incidence of previous sickling episodes
- The symptoms of current problems
  —infection
  —dehydration
  —crisis
- The presence of pre-existing organ damage
  —hepatic
  —renal
  —cardiorespiratory
  —skeletal
    -osteomyelitis
    -avascular necrosis

Examination. As part of the examination particular attention should be paid to:

- Cardiovascular system
  —blood pressure
  —ease of venous access
  —state of hydration

- Respiratory system
  —potential airway difficulties
  —evidence of infection

Investigation. The results of the following should be sought:

- Full blood count
- Haematocrit
- Reticulocyte count
- Blood film for the presence of sickle cells
- Haemoglobin electrophoresis
  —type of haemoglobin HbS, HbSC, HbS-β Thal
  —percentage HbA – increased risk of sickling if <25%
- Biochemistry
  —electrolytes, creatinine and urea
  —liver function tests

Management of labour and delivery. The principles of management are prevention of sickling during labour and delivery by avoiding hypoxia, hypotension, dehydration and infection. Haematocrit is maintained at 0.35–0.4 and the percentage of HbA at >50% by transfusion throughout the later stages of pregnancy.

Parturients with sickle cell trait (HbAS) usually have an uneventful peripartum period but it is prudent to avoid hypoxia and hypotension.

Analgesia for labour and vaginal delivery. Extradural analgesia is advised but care should be taken to avoid hypotension and stagnation and therefore sickling which may occur in the deep venous system of the lower limbs despite the increased blood flow to the skin.

In circumstances where extradural analgesia is contra-indicated parenteral opiates (pethidine 0.5–1 mg/kg i.v./i.m.) supplemented with Entonox are suitable alternatives.

Operative delivery. Regional techniques are recommended but care should be taken to maintain adequate hydration and avoid hypotension.

Where general anaesthesia is required no particular drugs confer any advantage but measures should be taken to:

- Give prophylactic antibiotics
- Pre-oxygenate for 5 minutes
- Increase FiO_2 to keep $SaO_2 > 95\%$
- Maintain $HbA > 50\%$
- Avoid hypothermia
- Ensure complete reversal of muscle relaxants
- Extubate the patient awake
- Give supplemental oxygen post-operatively for first 24 hours
- Ensure good post-operative analgesia

Regional anaesthesia in obstetrics

Introduction

The risks in the obstetric patient of difficulty of tracheal intubation, aspiration of gastric contents and awareness mean that general anaesthesia should be avoided wherever possible. Regional anaesthesia is relatively safe and the most effective means of providing analgesia during labour and operative delivery and enables the anaesthetist to avoid general anaesthesia in most instances.

The anaesthetist working on the labour ward is frequently asked to see a woman who is not sure whether she would like extradural analgesia for labour or for delivery by caesarean section. The purpose of this section is to provide an *aide memoire* so that an anaesthetist may be able to discuss the relative advantages and disadvantages of regional analgesia and allow the mother to come to an informed decision.

Later in the section some of the problems associated with regional anaesthesia in obstetrics and their management are described.

Anatomy and physiology

The pain pathways requiring block to provide analgesia and anaesthesia varies with the stage of labour and the operative procedure:

Labour
First stage – T10, **11, 12,** L1 roots – uterine contraction and dilation of cervix.
Second stage – The above plus roots S2, 3, 4 – distension of cervix, vagina, vulva and perineum.

Operative procedures
Cervical cerclage – T10 to S5
Forceps delivery – T10 to S5
Caesarean section – T4 to S5
Removal of retained placenta – T8 to S5

In current anaesthetic practice the two techniques most commonly used are extradural and subarachnoid blocks.

The use of subarachnoid catheters has not gained popularity in the UK and so subarachnoid block is not used to provide analgesia in labour.

The main aim is to produce sensory block but subarachnoid and extradural techniques may also cause motor and sympathetic block often leading to weakness, vasodilation, bradycardia and hypotension.

The place of regional anaesthesia in obstetrics is summarized in the following lists of indications and contraindications.

Indications
- Pain
- Uterine dysfunction
- Trial of labour or prolonged labour
- Systemic disease
    —cardiorespiratory
    —cerebrovascular
    —diabetes
    —pre-eclampsia
- Difficult intubation
- Instrumental delivery
- Prematurity of fetus and intrauterine growth retardation (IUGR)
- Breech presentation
- Multiple pregnancy

Contraindications
- Patient refusal
- Lack of immediately available anaesthetist
- Lack of experienced midwifery staff and resuscitation equipment
- Hypovolaemia and other fixed cardiac output states
- Local sepsis
- Bleeding diathesis or anticoagulated patient
- Gross spinal deformity – previous spinal surgery is not a contraindication unless it makes performance of the block technically difficult

32

The usual regional anaesthetic technique used during labour is lumbar extradural block maintained either by intermittent boluses or continuous infusion of local anaesthetic solutions with or without added opioids via an indwelling extradural catheter.

Extradural analgesia for labour and operative delivery

Extradural analgesia offers benefits to the parturient but the technique is not without complications. The advantages and disadvantages of extradural analgesia comprise:

Advantages
- It is the most effective analgesia available
- A reduced incidence of maternal and fetal acidosis
- The avoidance of side effects of opiates on mother and fetus
  - respiratory depression
  - sedation
  - nausea/vomiting
  - effect on gastric emptying
- It facilitates pain free vaginal examination, fetal blood sampling, and obstetric manipulation
- An improvement of placental blood flow

Disadvantages
- Requires special training of anaesthetist and midwife
- Need for intravenous line
- Relative immobility
- Risk of possible complications
  - hypotension – 10% with intravenous pre-load
  - backache – 15% – no different from patients without extradural

—headache – 70% – after inadvertent dural puncture
                8–25% – whatever the method of analgesia
—neurological damage – 1:100 000 incidence of permanent
  damage
- Prolongation of the second stage of labour
- Potential for increased incidence of forceps delivery

When considering the advantages of regional anaesthetic techniques to provide anaesthesia for operative procedures and manipulations one must compare regional anaesthesia with general anaesthesia as well as the advantages of one regional technique over another.

A comparison of regional anaesthesia and general anaesthesia for operative delivery

Advantages of regional anaesthesia
- Allows an awake mother
- Avoids the potential problems of airway management
- Minimizes the risk of maternal aspiration
- Precludes the possibility of inadvertent maternal awareness under light general anaesthesia
- Enables the participation of mother and father in delivery allowing early breast feeding and bonding
- Provides improved post-operative analgesia
- Reduces blood loss
- Leads to a better rate and quality of post-operative recovery
- Improves the condition of neonate

Disadvantages
- A slow onset of extradural block
- Occasional inadequate anaesthesia
- It is contraindicated in hypovolaemia and blood loss
- Possible hypotension
- The risk of neurological damage
- Possible urinary retention
- An incidence of headache following dural puncture

Table 2.1 A comparison of subarachnoid versus extradural block for operative delivery

Subarachnoid block	Extradural block
Advantages	
Technically easier	Should avoid dural puncture
Rapid onset (5 vs 20 mins)	Slower onset of hypotension
More intense block	Catheter technique allows flexibility
Dense motor block	in extent and duration of block
Small dose of local anaesthetic	
Disadvantages	
Rapid onset of hypotension	Larger dose of local anaesthetic and
Dural puncture headache	higher risk of high blocks and
	toxic reactions
Single dose technique:	Increased risk of inadequate height
limited duration	and quality of block
inflexible	

- The risk of toxic reaction to local anaesthetics because of the large doses used for extradural block
- Shivering which can be uncomfortable

The relative merits of subarachnoid and extradural blocks in providing anaesthesia for operative procedures are summarized below (Table 2.1).

In the remaining chapters of this section we will describe the complications of regional anaesthesia and their management.

Inadequate extradural analgesia

The quality of extradural analgesia during labour is a subjective assessment by the parturient of the whole period during which the extradural is in situ, and cannot be judged by an anaesthetist assessing the extent of anaesthesia at any one instant during labour. For example if top-ups are provided too infrequently the parturient may experience only intermittent pain relief throughout her labour, which she may consider unsatisfactory.

The incidence of complete failure of extradural block is 1% with inadequate block occurring in less than 5% of patients.

Features of a block which may lead to inadequate analgesia
- Missed segment
- Unilateral block
- Persistent sacral/rectal/lower back pain
- Complete failure

Assessment of block. If asked to review a mother who complains of inadequate analgesia check:

- Site and nature (continuous or intermittent) of pain
- Record of insertion
  - —site of catheter insertion
  - —length of catheter inserted and remaining in situ
  - —dose, time, and effect of first and subsequent doses of local anaesthetic
- The presence and extent of sympathetic block (vasodilation)
- Assess sensory block by means of assessing the loss of cold sensation to ethyl chloride spray
- Distension of the bladder – a potential cause of persistent suprapubic pain
- The progress of labour

The features of an inadequate extradural block and its management are summarized in Table 2.2.

If at the time of assessment delivery is judged to be imminent then further local anaesthetic is unnecessary, but an alternative such as Entonox should be offered.

It is important when performing any block to advise the mother of the risk of inadequate block. When performing a block for caesarean section the anaesthetist should record the height of block attained and the mother's satisfaction with the

Table 2.2 Management of inadequate extradural analgesia

Quality of block	Signs and symptoms	Action
Total failure	Absence of sensory or sympathetic block 20 minutes after dose of local anaesthetic	Re-site catheter
Inadequate height	Lower abdominal pain, bilateral sympathetic block with bilateral sensory block below dermatomal level of pain	Give additional dose of local anaesthetic (5 ml boluses of 0.25% bupivacaine)
Missed segment	Pain limited to discrete area (often groin), bilateral sympathetic and sensory block with discrete area of absence of sensory block	Give 5 ml of 2% lignocaine or 0.5% bupivacaine with patient on painful side If unsuccessful repeat after withdrawing catheter 1–2 cm If unsuccessful resite catheter
Unilateral block	Unilateral pain, sympathetic and sensory block	Withdraw catheter 1–2 cm and give 10 ml 2% lignocaine or 0.5% bupivacaine with parturient on painful side If unsuccessful resite catheter
Sacral or rectal pain	Sacral/lower back pain or pressure, bilateral sympathetic and sensory block not extending to sacral segments	Exclude occipito-posterior position or imminent delivery, give 10 ml of 2% lignocaine or 0.5% bupivacaine in sitting position
Full bladder	Persistent suprapubic pain with bilateral sympathetic and sensory block	Empty bladder by passing a catheter if necessary

37

block. If the block is inadequate then she should be offered general anaesthesia and her response recorded in the records. This should avoid the possibility of successful legal action against the anaesthetist.

Extensive block

Several causes of extensive block are described: total spinal anaesthesia, high spinal or extradural anaesthesia, and subdural (massive extradural injection). All share the common feature of extensive sensory block but differ in their speed of onset, motor block, incidence of hypotension and effect on consciousness.

Total spinal block.   The very rapid onset of hypotension, bradycardia, high sensory block, extensive paralysis, respiratory failure, and finally loss of consciousness with dilated pupils. The cause is the extensive cephalad spread of local anaesthetic within the subarachnoid space to the brain. This may be due to an overdose of local anaesthetic during spinal anaesthesia or more commonly the inadvertent injection of an extradural dose into the subarachnoid space during attempted extradural anaesthesia. Such injections may occur during the first injection through a Tuohy needle which has punctured the dura during insertion or during subsequent top-up injections through an extradural catheter which was either incorrectly placed or has migrated into the subarachnoid space.

Significance.   The hypotension and respiratory failure associated with total spinal block have obvious deleterious effects on maternal and fetal well-being. Provided the event is immediately recognized and promptly managed, no harm should come to either mother or fetus.

Management. The aims of management are: protection of the airway, management of both respiratory failure and hypotension.

In the event of suspected total spinal block the following actions should be instituted:

- Summon senior assistance and the obstetric team
- Position mother in the wedged position with a slight head-down tilt. This will prevent aortocaval compression, provide an autotransfusion from the lower limbs and may limit cephalad spread of local anaesthetic, if the solution is hypobaric relative to CSF
- Assess airway, respiration and vital signs
- Give 100% oxygen by mask, ventilate with bag and mask prior to intubation. Remember cricoid pressure should be used if the mother cannot protect her airway
- Treat hypotension with intravenous crystalloid solutions and increments of ephedrine (15 mg i.v. with the same dose i.m.) and repeat as necessary
- Monitor maternal vital signs and fetal heart rate
- If the fetus is compromised, delivery should be expedited. If however maternal and fetal signs are stable the above management should continue until the block regresses spontaneously (2–4 hours)
- In the event of maternal cardiac arrest (q.v.) full cardio-pulmonary resuscitation (CPR) should be instituted and delivery of the fetus may be necessary to permit successful resuscitation of the mother

High spinal anaesthesia. There is a rapid onset of sensory and motor block with associated hypotension as with total spinal block. The extent of the block is not so extensive and as the local anaesthetic does not reach the brain stem there is no loss of consciousness. If the local anaesthetic reaches the upper cervical segments then respiratory inadequacy is likely.

Management. The treatment of a high spinal block relies on careful monitoring of the parturient's vital signs, treatment of hypotension and respiratory insufficiency as described, as well as careful explanation and reassurance.

Subdural or 'massive' extradural block. This follows the unintentional injection of local anaesthetic into the subdural extra-arachnoid space. It is the postulated mechanism for the unusual sequelae following the injection of an extradural (10–15 ml) dose of local anaesthetic, which include; slow onset (15–20 min); extensive sensory block; limited motor block; progressive but slow respiratory failure and recovery within 2 hours. Significant hypotension is rarely a feature of this condition.

Management. The management of a subdural block involves the principles of cardiorespiratory support described above.

Bloody tap

Definition. A bloody tap is the puncture of an extradural vein by a Tuohy needle or catheter.

Physiological significance. The chances of puncturing extradural veins are increased during pregnancy because of the engorged state of the extradural venous plexus, especially during a uterine contraction.

The dangers of extradural vein puncture are:

- The possibility of intravenous injection of local anaesthetic and toxicity (q.v.)
- Extradural haematoma (q.v.) formation

Prevention and management. The risks of vessel puncture are reduced by avoiding insertion of the Tuohy needle during uterine contraction.

Vessel puncture or cannulation by Tuohy needle or catheter can be verified by gentle aspiration and the use of an adrenaline containing solution for the 'test dose', but neither of these provide 100% confirmation.

In the event of a bloody tap or suspected intravenous placement of either Tuohy needle or catheter they should be withdrawn and the extradural space located at an adjacent interspace.

Toxic reaction to local anaesthetics

Definition. Systemic toxicity occurs when the plasma level of local anaesthetic reaches a level which causes disturbance of the central nervous and cardiovascular systems by stabilizing their excitable membranes.

The plasma level of local anaesthetic achieved depends on:

- Total dose = concentration × volume
- Rate of injection
- Site of injection
- Addition of vasoconstrictors

The toxicity of each local anaesthetic is different and is related to:

- The potency of the agent for neural block
- The lipid solubility of the agent
- The degree of binding of the local anaesthetic to myocardial proteins

Diagnosis. The brain is more sensitive to the effects of local anaesthetics than the myocardium so that the first manifestations of systemic toxicity are the responses of the central nervous system (CNS) and only later the cardiovascular system.

The initial excitatory symptoms, e.g. seizures, are caused by the initial block of inhibitory neurones and as levels of drug rise, generalized depression of the central nervous system occurs.

Signs and symptoms of central nervous system toxicity:
- Numbness of tongue and mouth
- Lightheadedness
- Tinnitus
- Visual disturbance
- Inappropriate behaviour
- Drowsiness/unconsciousness
- Slurred speech
- Muscle twitching
- Convulsions
- Apnoea

Because of the relative resistance of the cardiovascular system, clinical signs of myocardial toxicity are seen at levels 2–4 times those causing convulsions.

Signs of cvs toxicity:
- Hypotension
- Bradycardia
- Arrhythmias
- Cardiac arrest – bupivacaine often causes arrest in ventricular fibrillation

Physiological significance.   Without urgent treatment of convulsions, apnoea and/or cardiac arrest there is a likelihood of maternal and fetal hypoxia and acidosis which if untreated will lead to irreversible hypoxic brain damage.

Prevention and treatment

Prevention.   Bearing in mind that the commonest causes of systemic toxicity are intravascular injection or absolute overdosage of drug, the risk of toxicity can be minimized by applying these rules:

1. Do not exceed the maximum recommended dose of a particular local anaesthetic (see Table 2.3).

Table 2.3 Recommended maximum doses of the commonly used local anaesthetics

	Recommended maximum dose (mg/kg)
Bupivacaine plain	2
Bupivacaine plus adrenaline	4
Lignocaine plain	3
Lignocaine plus adrenaline	7

2. Aspirate gently before injecting to exclude intravascular placement of the needle or catheter.
3. Inject the dose slowly.
4. When administering large doses of local anaesthetic inject the total dose in increments.

Treatment. When performing regional blocks ensure that resuscitation equipment and drugs are available. The anaesthetist should remember that there are two patients, mother and fetus and both should be monitored throughout the treatment period.

When the diagnosis of a toxic reaction is made:

1. Summon the assistance of anaesthetic, obstetric and midwifery staff.
2. Ensure a clear airway and give 100% oxygen by face mask initially. This may be all that is required in a mild reaction. Positive pressure ventilation may be required if the mother is apnoeic.
3. If convulsions occur:
    —place mother head down in the wedged position to avoid aspiration and aortocaval compression
    —treat with incremental doses of diazepam (5–10 mg) or thiopentone (25–50 mg)
    —monitor maternal vital signs and the fetal heart rate
    —if the airway is compromised tracheal intubation is indicated. This may be facilitated by suxamethonium and cricoid pressure should be used.

4.   If cardiovascular collapse is a feature of the reaction:
    —treat hypotension with ephedrine (15–30 mg) i.v. which
    has vasoconstrictor (alpha receptor-agonist) and myo-
    cardial stimulant (beta receptor-agonist) effects, and i.v.
    fluids (1000 ml Hartmann's solution). Further con-
    tinuous infusion of inotropes may be required e.g.
    dobutamine 5–15 mcg/kg/min which can be given via a
    peripheral line
    —monitor fetal well-being. If its condition is satisfactory
    postpone delivery until the local anaesthetic levels
    subside and the mother's condition stabilizes. If it is in
    jeopardy immediate delivery is indicated and the pae-
    diatricians should be informed
    —if cardiac arrest occurs full cardiopulmonary resuscita-
    tion should be instituted (cf. cardiac arrest in
    pregnancy).

Management of bupivacaine cardiotoxicity.   Bupivacaine toxicity causes specific difficulties of resuscitation. The affinity of
bupivacaine for myocardial tissue, increased toxicity in acido-
tic tissues and a tendency to produce ventricular fibrillation
cause cardiovascular collapse which is resistant to the usual
supportive therapy.
Treatment includes:

• Prolonged cardiopulmonary support
• Early correction of acidosis
• i.v. bretylium loading dose 5–10 mg/kg, maintenance
  1–2 mg/min – to treat ventricular fibrillation that is resistant
  to DC cardioversion
• High doses of inotropes e.g. dobutamine (10–20 µg/kg/min)
  or adrenaline (0.01–0.1 µg/kg/min)

Urinary retention

Retention of urine can occur during and after labour. It is more common following extradural or spinal anaesthesia or instrumental delivery. Central blocks often require the liberal use of intravenous fluids which increases urine production. The block also reduces bladder sensation, making the parturient unaware of a full bladder for up to 48 hours post delivery.

Other causes of urinary retention include:

- Pain
- Retroverted uterus
- Faecal impaction
- Hypotonic bladder
- Pre-existing neurological deficit

Significance. Bladder distension as a result of retention may lead to:

- Persistent suprapubic pain following institution of extradural block
- Prevention of fetal descent
- Damage to the bladder during delivery

Management. During labour a parturient with an extradural in situ should be encouraged to micturate before each top-up. If an extradural infusion is being used during labour or after delivery the parturient is asked to attempt to micturate every 3–4 hours, which is often possible despite anaesthesia. When this regimen is unsuccessful they should have sterile catheterization as required. The incidence of urinary tract infection is lower after repeated catheterization than with an indwelling catheter.

In most centres mothers having caesarean section are catheterized routinely and the catheter left in place post-operatively.

Dural puncture headache

Definition. Dural puncture headache is the characteristic headache following the perforation of the dura, intentionally during spinal block or accidentally while attempting to locate the extradural space.

The mechanism behind the development of symptoms is the leak of CSF through a tear in the dura causing a reduction in CSF pressure and therefore traction on the pain sensitive structures around the brain.

Diagnosis. The features of the headache are:

- *Onset:* any time up to 3 days post puncture
- *Site:* occipital or occasionally frontal
- *Radiation:* neck, shoulders and extending over the vertex
- *Exacerbating/relieving factors:* worse on standing, sitting, straining; relieved by supine position and abdominal compression
- *Severity:* incapacitating
- *Associated features:*
  —neck stiffness
  —nausea/vomiting
  —photophobia
  —cranial nerve palsies especially the VIth nerve
  —tinnitus
  —hypoacusis
- *Duration:* if untreated, from days to several weeks

Incidence. Related to the size, shape and number of holes in the dura

18G Tuohy needle, 70%
26G spinal needle, 3–6%
29G spinal needle, 1–2%
24G pencil point needle, 1–2%

46

Management. As prophylaxis against the development of dural puncture headache use small diameter or pencil point spinal needles when performing subarachnoid blocks.

But in the event of confirmed *accidental* dural puncture treatment should comprise:

1. Immediate withdrawal of the Tuohy needle or catheter. Insertion of another extradural catheter in an adjacent interspace and ensure effective analgesia is achieved.
2. following delivery infusion of 1–1.5 l of N-saline into extradural space via the extradural catheter over 24 hours to increase extradural pressure.

If asked to see a mother complaining of headache in the postpartum period management should include:

- *History* – take a full history to exclude other causes of headache. Most are minor, but subdural haematoma has been described as a complication of dural puncture
- *Reassurance* – reassure the mother that any headache will resolve eventually even without therapy
- *Hydration* – maintain good hydration (3 l of fluid per day)
- *Posture* – enforced recumbency has no effect on the incidence or duration of headache but offers symptomatic relief
- *Laxatives* – give laxatives to prevent straining at stool
- *Symptomatic relief* – use simple analgesics: paracetamol, NSAIDs and if necessary codeine phosphate (1 mg/kg p.o./i.m.)
- *'Blood patch'* – if the headache has not resolved within 2 days the use of an extradural autologous 'blood patch' should be recommended to the patient

Extradural 'blood patch'. 10–15 ml of the patients blood is collected under strict aseptic conditions, and injected slowly into the extradural space at the level of the dural puncture. The injection should be painless, if not the position of the needle should be adjusted. The blood patch is successful in 90% of cases. If unsuccessful or the headache recurs a second patch may be performed.

Shivering

Shivering is the involuntary episodic clonic contraction of skeletal muscle. It is a well recognized complication of extradural block occurring in approximately 10% of blocks. The aetiology of the phenomenon is thought to be due to stimulation of temperature sensitive receptors in the extradural space.

Physiological significance. Shivering causes an increase in oxygen consumption upto three times resting rates of consumption but this rarely results in maternal hypoxia.

The associated increase in cardiac output makes additional demands on the maternal cardiovascular system and the release of catecholamines can reduce placental blood flow and lead to fetal acidosis.

For the mother shivering can be very uncomfortable and cause marked distress which may have an adverse effect on placental blood flow.

Prevention and management. Several measures can be taken to prevent and treat shivering caused by extradural block.

The intravenous fluids given as pre-load prior to administration of local anaesthetic should be thoroughly warmed to body temperature. The same applies to the local anaesthetic solutions before injection into the extradural space.

If shivering occurs despite these measures then opioids can be mixed with the local anaesthetic solutions. Give 25 µg of fentanyl with the next top-up dose.

Broken extradural catheter

This is a very rare complication of extradural block.

Causes. Shearing may occur if a catheter is withdrawn through the needle, when it is sheared by the bevel. Vigorous attempts to remove a catheter which has become stuck because of kinking, knotting or being pinched between two vertebrae, may also lead to breakage of the catheter.

Prevention. Catheters should not be withdrawn through Tuohy needles. If necessary both needle and catheter should be withdrawn together.

Flexion of the spine may be needed to release a catheter that has become stuck.

Management. Broken catheters have been left in situ without complication because of the inert and sterile nature of extradural catheters. The difficulty of locating fragments in the extradural space (catheters are no more radio-opaque than bone), makes attempts at surgical removal ill advised. The patient and her GP should be informed and reassured and further treatment is unnecessary unless new symptoms and signs develop.

Prolonged neurological deficit

The parturients' greatest fear of regional anaesthesia is neurological damage.

In obstetrics extradural anaesthesia is one of several possible causes of neurological damage, all fortunately rare. Features of these causes and their likely outcome are summarized in Table 2.4.

Accurate early diagnosis and treatment is important and may require the involvement of a neurologist.

Table 2.4 Types of neurological damage following labour under extradural analgesia

Pathology	Cause	Onset	Features	Outcome
Spinal nerve neuropathy	Trauma to nerve by needle or catheter	0–2 days	Pain on insertion of needle or catheter and on injection Pain, paraesthesia and numbness in distribution of nerve	Recovery in 1–12 weeks
Peripheral nerve palsies	Trauma from instrumental delivery and compression caused by poor positioning of parturient	Hours	Motor and sensory loss in distribution of affected nerves e.g. foot drop	Recovery 1–12 weeks
Adhesive arachnoiditis	Irritant injectate, e.g. incorrect or contaminated solutions	Immediate	Pain on injection variable deficit Painful, progressive paraplegia	Progressive painful disability
Extradural haematoma or abscess	Spontaneous, coagulopathy bacteraemia	0–4 days	Backache and progressive paraplegia	Urgent surgical intervention to prevent permanent paraplegia
Prolonged effect of local anaesthetic	Repeated dose of high concentration of local anaesthetic	Hours	Sensory +/– motor loss in distribution of spinal root	Recovery in days

Extradural haematoma and abscess

Extradural haematoma

Definition. An extradural haematoma is a collection of blood in the extradural space. It may occur spontaneously, but is more common following extradural vessel puncture, especially in the presence of a coagulopathy or anticoagulant therapy. It behaves as a space occupying lesion in the spinal canal causing compression damage to the spinal cord or cauda equina.

Diagnosis. The earliest symptom is the sudden onset of severe pain in the back and the development of a neurological deficit. The presence of concomitant sensory block from local anaesthetics may mask the pain and can make the diagnosis difficult.

Extradural abscess

Definition. An extradural abscess is a collection of pus in the extradural space which has similar effects to a haematoma.
   An extradural abscess may arise from septicaemia or be due to secondary infection of an extradural haematoma formed during the performance of an extradural block.

Diagnosis. Symptoms and signs classically develop 3–4 days after the insertion of an extradural, and include localized tenderness over the spine, signs and symptoms of infection and progressive and persistent neurological deficit.

Management. Extradural haematoma or abscess may cause compression of the spinal cord or cauda equina and require urgent evacuation to prevent permanent neurological damage.

The possibility of extradural haematoma makes it vital that the regression of any central block is monitored and recorded.

In the event of a suspected extradural haematoma or abscess the urgent involvement of senior anaesthetic, radiological and neurosurgical personnel is indicated to confirm the diagnosis and arrange for the evacuation of the haematoma or abscess and the initiation of antibiotic therapy.

Emergencies

Cardiac Arrest

The incidence of cardiac arrest in pregnancy is low (1:30 000 pregnancies). Several physiological and anatomical changes of late pregnancy make resuscitation of the mother difficult.

External cardiac compression is difficult because of breast enlargement, raised diaphragm, obesity and splayed ribs. The rate of compression needs to be higher than usual because of the increased cardiac output of pregnancy (40%).

Vena caval compression by the gravid uterus may make resuscitation impossible by preventing venous return and aortic compression by the same mechanism will further compromise fetal outcome.

The securing of a clear airway particularly by tracheal intubation is made difficult by complete dentition; short, thick neck; enlarged breasts and the presence of gastric contents which are more likely to be regurgitated by the gravid mother.

Ventilation is more difficult to achieve and assess because of the detrimental effects of obesity and splinting of the diaphragm on chest compliance.

Because of these factors it is important that all members of the obstetric team – midwife, obstetrician and anaesthetist – are familiar with the problems of resuscitation and receive regular refresher courses in basic and advanced life support (BLS and ALS) of the pregnant woman.

Diagnosis. The absence of a pulse in a major blood vessel (carotid or femoral) is diagnostic of cardiac arrest but other features should suggest the diagnosis:

- Sudden loss of consciousness
- Cyanosis and abnormal or absent respirations
- Asystole, ventricular fibrillation or ventricular tachycardia on the ECG
- Unrecordable blood pressure

Physiological significance. Absence of cardiac output results in the cessation of blood flow to vital organs leading to tissue hypoxia and acidosis and vital organ failure. Prolonged acidosis causes vasodilation and unresponsiveness of the cardiovascular system to catecholamines.

Irreversible brain damage occurs after 3-4 minutes of anoxia in the non-pregnant patient but in late pregnancy oxygen consumption is increased (20%) thus reducing this margin of safety.

For the fetus, maternal cardiac arrest has a direct and immediate effect on placental blood flow. Although the fetus is able to survive more prolonged periods of hypoxia than the mother, its survival depends on a resumption of maternal cardiac output or urgent delivery and conversion to an extrauterine circulation.

Causes of cardiac arrest

Primary causes relating directly to disease of the heart
- Myocardial ischaemia
- Cardiomyopathy
- Aortic valve disease

Secondary causes
- Hypoxaemia following aspiration of gastric contents; failed intubation; inadvertent oesophageal intubation; airway obstruction; hypoventilation; hypoxic gas mixtures; or low cardiac output
- Hypovolaemia usually from utero-placental haemorrhage but it may also be secondary to cerebrovascular haemorrhage associated with pre-eclampsia
- Hypotension caused by vena caval compression, anaphylaxis, vasodilating drugs, e.g. anti-hypertensives and regional anaesthesia
- Myocardial depression by drugs such as general anaesthetic agents, local anaesthetic agents injected intravenously or cardioactive drugs used in the management of pre-eclampsia, e.g. β-blockers or calcium antagonists
- Pulmonary or amniotic embolism

Management. The management of a cardiac arrest in the labour ward or other hospital setting involves the following:

- Confirm diagnosis
- Put in wedged position with uterus displaced
- Commence basic life support (BLS)
- Summon obstetric team, with equipment and drugs for advanced life support (ALS)
- Initiate ALS
- Proceed to caesarean section if no response to the above within 5 minutes
- Consider open cardiac massage if no progress is made
- If resuscitation is successful arrange transfer to intensive therapy unit for:
  —cardiovascular monitoring and support
  —respiratory support
  —cerebral resuscitation

Basic life support

Airway – clear of dentures, vomitus and foreign bodies, and perform jaw thrust

Breathing – commence intermittent positive pressure ventilation by bag and mask with 100% oxygen, if ventilation allows apply cricoid pressure until cuffed tracheal tube inserted and position confirmed by auscultation or capnography.

Circulation – single resuscitator – external cardiac compression at 80–100/minute with two breaths given every 15 compressions, two resuscitators – one breath every 5 compressions.

Advanced life support. When the appropriate equipment arrives at the scene of the arrest resuscitation should proceed to ALS including *intubation*, continued *external cardiac compression*, interrupted only for *defibrillation*, and the administration of *drugs* (see Figure 3.1).

Problems in Obstetric Anaesthesia

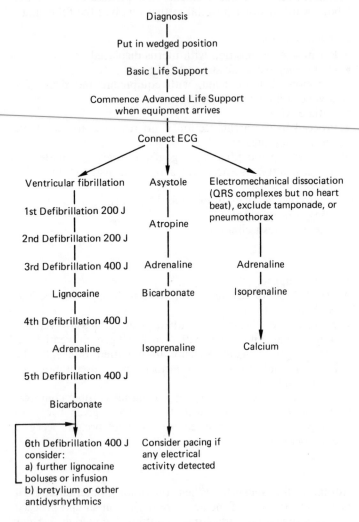

Diagnosis

Put in wedged position

Basic Life Support

Commence Advanced Life Support
when equipment arrives

Connect ECG

Ventricular fibrillation

1st Defibrillation 200 J

2nd Defibrillation 200 J

3rd Defibrillation 400 J

Lignocaine

4th Defibrillation 400 J

Adrenaline

5th Defibrillation 400 J

Bicarbonate

6th Defibrillation 400 J
consider:
a) further lignocaine
boluses or infusion
b) bretylium or other
antidysrhythmics

Asystole

Atropine

Adrenaline

Bicarbonate

Isoprenaline

Consider pacing if
any electrical
activity detected

Electromechanical dissociation
(QRS complexes but no heart
beat), exclude tamponade, or
pneumothorax

Adrenaline

Isoprenaline

Calcium

Figure 3.1 Cardiopulmonary resuscitation in pregnancy.

Intubation should be performed with consideration for the anticipated anatomical and physiological changes associated with late pregnancy (see above), and may be facilitated by correct positioning of the patient with neck flexed and head extended on the neck.

Haemorrhage

Haemorrhage in the peripartum period is a significant source of maternal and fetal morbidity and mortality.

Definition

Antepartum haemorrhage. This is vaginal blood loss after the 24th week of pregnancy. It can be expected to occur in just less than 5% of pregnancies.

Postpartum haemorrhage. This is blood loss of >500 ml in the first 24 hours of the postpartum period. It occurs in 5% of pregnancies.

Physiological significance. Blood loss has obvious effects on circulating blood volume. A reduction in blood volume will reduce cardiac output and a fall in blood pressure will occur unless compensatory changes in the cardiovascular system are initiated. These include an increase in heart rate and myocardial contractility and vasoconstriction. A significant proportion (10%) of total maternal cardiac output goes to the placenta but there is little or no autoregulatory capacity in the placental circulation and so placental perfusion is directly proportional to maternal blood pressure. Maternal hypotension secondary to antepartum haemorrhage will have obvious detrimental implications for fetal gas exchange leading to hypoxaemia and metabolic acidosis.

Loss of red blood cells will reduce the oxygen carrying capacity of the circulation and with a reduction in cardiac output will lead to a fall in oxygen supply to the fetus and maternal vital organs.

Cardiac output = [Heart rate × Stroke volume]
Oxygen content of blood = [Haemoglobin × SaO_2 × 1.39]

Oxygen flow = Cardiac output × Oxygen content of blood

In the non-pregnant state a patient may tolerate acute loss of 20% of circulating blood volume before requiring blood transfusion providing loss is replaced with crystalloid or colloid. Because of the 35% increase in circulating blood volume induced by pregnancy a pregnant woman at term may tolerate up to 30% loss of circulating volume without incurring a fall in haematocrit. Despite this it is important to remember that anaemia of pregnancy may result in haemoglobin levels at term of <10 g% indicating the need for earlier blood transfusion.

Aetiology.   In both the antepartum and postpartum periods haemorrhage may be either revealed and lost per vagina, or concealed within the uterus and pelvis.

Causes of antepartum haemorrhage

Revealed:
- Abruptio placenta
- Placenta praevia
- Rupture of vasa praevia
- Disorders of haemostasis (q.v.)

Concealed:
- Abruptio placenta – even large retroplacental collections may not be manifest as vaginal blood loss
- Uterine rupture
- Ruptured utero-ovarian vein

Causes of postpartum haemorrhage

Revealed:
- Birth canal trauma
- Uterine atony due to:
  —prolonged labour
  —multiple gestation
  —use of excessive volatile agent
  —abnormal uterine anatomy
- Uterine inversion (q.v.) or rupture
- Retained products of conception
- Coagulopathy

Concealed:
- Haematoma:
  —vulval
  —broad ligament
- Utero-ovarian vein rupture

There are several features which should make the obstetric team aware of the increased likelihood of postpartum haemorrhage:

- Previous antepartum haemorrhage
- Previous retained placenta
- Multiple fetuses
- Prolonged labour
- Operative delivery
- Abnormal uterine anatomy
- Coagulopathy

Management. Anyone working on an obstetric unit should be well versed and know their role in the management of the bleeding, pregnant woman. There should be: monitoring equipment; equipment for the rapid administration of warm intravenous fluid; ready availability of crystalloid and colloid intravenous fluids and prompt access to haematology and blood transfusion services.

When significant blood loss is suspected the following should be instituted:

1. Face mask oxygen
2. Establishment of good venous access – two large bore cannulae 14G or 16G and fluids given with the aid of pressurized infusors
3. Monitoring: ECG, non-invasive blood pressure, fetal heart rate (if appropriate), central venous pressure and urine output
4. Further anaesthetic and ancillary help should be summoned to help in resuscitation
5. Alert the haematology and transfusion service
6. A rapid assessment of severity of blood loss (Table 3.1) and the possible cause
7. Brief anaesthetic history and examination

Fluid therapy. Fluid therapy should be with crystalloid (Hartmann's) initially, which has the advantage of availability. Up to 20 ml/kg of crystalloid should be given and if blood is required but not yet available colloid solutions (Gelofusine, Hetastarch or Albumin) should be used in the interim. It should be remembered that volume replacement is more important than provision of red blood cells and colloid should not be stopped while waiting for blood.

If more than 20 ml/kg of colloid are required and blood loss continues, emergency O Rh-negative blood should be used if the arrival of crossmatched blood is not imminent.

While resuscitation is initiated the cause of the blood loss should be established and treated. General anaesthesia (q.v.) may be required to establish the diagnosis or to treat the cause of haemorrhage. Regional anaesthesia is contraindicated in the presence of hypovolaemia.

General anaesthesia should involve a rapid sequence technique following pre-oxygenation and application of cricoid pressure.

Induction with etomidate (0.2–0.3 mg/kg) or ketamine (1–2 mg/kg i.v.) may be indicated in the hypovolaemic patient. Volatile agents are poorly tolerated in hypovolaemia and a

Table 3.1 Pathophysiological changes of blood loss

	Upto 15%	15–30%	% Total blood volume loss 30–40%	>40%
Volume blood loss	Upto 750 ml	750–1500 ml	1500–2000 ml	>2000 ml
Heart rate	<100	>100	>120	>140
Systolic blood pressure	>100 mmHg	<100 mmHg	<90 mmHg	<80 mmHg
Urine output	>30 ml/hr	20–30 ml/hr	5–15 ml/hr	<5 ml/hr
Capillary refill	<2 seconds	>2 seconds	>2 seconds	>2 seconds
Respiratory rate	15–20	20–30	30–40	>40
Mental state	Anxious	Anxious	Anxious and confused	Obtunded

relaxant nitrous oxide/oxygen combination may be justified until intravascular volume has been restored. Minimal concentrations of volatile agent should be used in all cases of haemorrhage except for retained placenta where relaxation of the uterus may be necessary to allow the obstetrician to perform a manual removal of the placenta.

Once general anaesthesia has been achieved the anaesthetist is free to:

- Connect warming coils to i.v. fluid giving sets
- Insert central venous and intra-arterial cannulae
- Arrange insertion of urinary catheter
- Send specimens for haematocrit and clotting screen to assess the effects of resuscitation and exclude a coagulopathy

Assessment of resuscitation. The aim of therapy is the maintenance of tissue oxygenation. Adequate resuscitation is indicated by:

- Heart rate <100 bpm
- Systolic blood pressure >100 mmHg
- Central venous pressure 5–10 cmH$_2$O
- Urine output >0.5 ml/kg/hour
- Capillary refill time <2 seconds

Haemostatic failure

Pregnancy causes marked changes in the mother's haemostatic mechanisms:

- Increase in Factors II, V, VII, VIII, X and fibrinogen
- Reduced antithrombin III
- Reduced fibrinolysis

Some complications of pregnancy, e.g. pre-eclampsia and DIC cause further deleterious derangement of the process.

The obstetric anaesthetist may be involved in the management of parturients with abnormalities of haemostasis. They should be aware of the implications for the management of analgesia and anaesthesia during labour and delivery.

Definition. Haemostatic failure is a disorder of any or all of the components of the normal haemostatic process:

- Vasoconstriction
- Platelet function
- Clotting factors

Aetiology. Disorders of haemostasis may be congenital or acquired.

Congenital:
- Von Willebrand's disease
- Symptomatic carriers of haemophilia A

Acquired:
- Platelet abnormalities
  —thrombocytopenia (reduced platelet numbers)
  - Pre-eclampsia
  - Drug-induced
  - Idiopathic thrombocytopenic purpura (ITP)
  - Thrombotic thrombocytopenic purpura (TTP)
  —thrombopathia (abnormal platelet function)
  - Aspirin therapy
  - Dypiridamole
- Clotting abnormalities
  —Disseminated intravascular coagulation (DIC)
  —Pre-eclampsia
  —Iatrogenic, i.e. heparin therapy
- Vascular abnormalities
  —Systemic lupus erythematosus (SLE)
  —Henoch-Schönlein purpura

Assessment of haemostatic failure

History.
- Bleeding or bruising in patient or their family
- Type of bleeding
  —vascular/platelet problems cause petechiae and purpura
  —clotting problems cause extensive bleeding with ecchymoses or haemarthroses

Examination. This should include the skin, mucosae, joints and optic fundi.

Investigations

Test	Significance	Normal value
Platelet count	Platelet plug formation	$150–400 \times 10^9/l$
Bleeding time		2–9 minutes
Activated partial thromboplastin time (aPTT)	Intrinsic pathway function	35–45 seconds
Prothrombin time (PT)	Extrinsic pathway function	12–14 seconds
Fibrinogen	Consumptive coagulopathy	2–5 g/l
Fibrin degradation products (FDP)	Excessive thrombolysis	<10 mg/l

Physiological significance

Mother. For mothers with a pre-existing haemostatic defect, pregnancy may cause a deterioration of the underlying cause, e.g. systemic lupus erythematosus (SLE) or idiopathic thrombocytopenic purpura (ITP).

The existence of haemostatic failure increases the danger of peripartum haemorrhage which may threaten both mother and fetus.

Regional anaesthesia is contraindicated in the presence of haemostatic failure because of the risk of extradural haematoma formation so the choice of analgesic techniques available to the mother is limited.

The anaesthetist must always be careful during laryngoscopy, intubation and extubation to avoid causing bleeding and upper airway obstruction.

Close observation during the post-operative period is recommended in case any haematoma produced later causes upper airway obstruction.

Fetus.   Maternal conditions causing haemostatic disturbance may lead to fetal loss.

The defect of haemostasis may be transmitted to the neonate, e.g. ITP and drug-induced thrombocytopenia.

Management.   The anaesthetic management of the parturient with a significant disturbance of haemostatic function requires an experienced anaesthetist and consultation with a haematologist. Table 3.2 summarizes the clinical features, changes in haemostasis, and the management of analgesia and anaesthesia for labour and delivery of the most frequently seen disturbances of haemostasis. For more detailed management regimens the reader is referred to more comprehensive texts.

Embolism

Definition.   Embolism is the sudden blocking of an artery by blood clot, foreign body or other material. Pulmonary embolism, the obstruction of the pulmonary arteries with blood clot, is the commonest source of embolism and is one of the most frequent causes of mortality in the obstetric

Table 3.2 Haemostatic defects during pregnancy

	Clinical features	Haemostatic tests	Analgesia for labour and normal vaginal delivery	Operative delivery
Platelet disorders				
(i) *Thrombocytopenia:* Drug induced, auto-immune (ITP, SLE)	Epistaxis, bleeding gums, ecchymoses Previous splenectomy Drug history	Platelet count reduced Bleeding time prolonged PT normal aPTT normal TT normal	Lumbar extradural contraindicated if platelets $<100 \times 10^9$/l or bleeding time prolonged >12 min. Give i.v. opiates supplemented with Entonox	General anaesthesia if regional blockade contraindicated Give platelets to keep platelet count >50 $\times$ 10^9/l
(ii) *Thrombopathia:* Aspirin therapy	History of consumption	Platelet count normal Bleeding time prolonged PT normal aPTT normal TT normal	As above	As above
(iii) *Pre-eclampsia*	Features of pre-eclampsia: hypertension oedema proteinuria	Platelet count normal or reduced Bleeding time normal or reduced PT normal aPTT normal TT normal Fibrin degradation products normal	As above	As above Delivery of placenta should reverse haemostatic derangement

Clotting abnormality

Hereditary

Clotting abnormality				
von Willebrand's disease	Mennorhagia Epistaxis Haemarthroses Excessive post traumatic/surgical bleeding may improve during pregnancy	Platelet count normal Bleeding time prolonged Mild 12–24 min Severe 30 min PT normal aPTT prolonged TT normal Factor VIII reduced	Extradural analgesia contraindicated Infiltration of the perineum with local anaesthetic is safe	General anaesthesia Factor VIII replacement for operative period Normal vaginal delivery: 30–40% activity Operative delivery: 80–100% activity
Haemophilia A carrier	See von Willebrands	Platelet count normal Bleeding time normal Mild 12–24 min Severe 30 min PT normal aPTT prolonged TT normal Factor VIII reduced	See von Willebrand's	See von Willebrand's
Acquired				
Anticoagulant therapy	Epistaxis, GI bleeding, ecchymoses usually secondary to heparin therapy	Platelet count normal or reduced Bleeding time normal PT normal or prolonged aPTT prolonged Activated clotting time (ACT) prolonged	Extradural analgesia contraindicated	General anaesthesia Reverse heparin with protamine 1 mg/100 units of heparin given

continued

69

Table 3.2 (*continued*)

	Clinical features	Haemostatic tests	Analgesia for labour and normal vaginal delivery	Operative delivery
Disseminated intravascular coagulopathy (DIC)	Bleeding in the presence of known precipitants of DIC: placental abruprothrombin timeion intrauterine death amniotic fluid embolism	Platelet count reduced PT normal aPTT normal TT prolonged Fibrinogen reduced FDP increased Red cell fragments on blood film	Extradural analgesia contraindicated	General anaesthesia Treatment of underlying cause
Vascular defect e.g. Systemic lupus (SLE)	Evidence of multisystem involvement: vasculitis purpura thrombosis arthropathy cardiac and cns symptoms	Platelet count reduced Bleeding time prolonged PT prolonged aPTT prolonged Circulating anticoagulant	Extradural analgesia usually safe if platelet count, bleeding time and clotting normal	General anaesthesia if regional blockade is contraindicated Give platelets if count <50 × 10⁹/l Steroid cover may be required

population. Amniotic fluid embolism is a rare but frequently fatal condition peculiar to pregnancy. Air embolism is a possible but rare complication of caesarean section and extradural analgesia.

Physiological significance. The lungs filter material from the systemic venous return and remove it from the circulation. When emboli of significant size or quantity become trapped in the pulmonary vascular bed there are physiological changes common to all embolic syndromes:

- Obstruction to pulmonary blood flow and pulmonary hypertension
- Right ventricular strain
- Cardiac failure
- Ventilation–perfusion mismatch due to shunting of blood through the lungs
- Hypoxia

Diagnosis and management

Pulmonary embolism. The obstetric patient is at particular risk of deep vein thrombosis and pulmonary embolism because of the relative immobility and hypercoagulable state of pregnancy and the frequency of pelvic surgery. Pulmonary embolism may occur at any time in the antepartum, peripartum or postpartum period.

Diagnosis. Features of pulmonary clot embolism include:

- Tachypnoea
- Pleuritic chest pain
- Hypoxia – unresponsive to increased FiO_2
- Tachycardia
- Hypotension
- ECG changes: tachydysrhythmias, $S_1Q_3T_3$, RV strain
- A sudden fall in end-tidal carbon dioxide tension
- An abnormal ventilation – perfusion scan
- Abnormal pulmonary angiogram

Management. The degree of therapeutic intervention depends on the clinical severity of the condition, but includes:

- Cardiovascular support with cardiac massage, fluids and inotropes to maintain right ventricular output
- Positive pressure ventilation to reduce the work of respiration
- Thrombolysis and anticoagulation
    —streptokinase: loading dose 250 000 u;
      maintenance dose 100 000 u/hour for 24 hours keeping thrombin time at >1.5 times control
    —heparin: bolus 5000 u, then 1000 u/hour to maintain the activated partial thromboplastin time at 2.5 times the normal
    —warfarin for long-term oral anticoagulation:
      loading dose 0.5 mg/kg then maintenance of 5–12 mg/day to keep the INR at 2.0–3.0
- Pulmonary thromboembolectomy (rarely practicable)

Amniotic fluid embolism. This occurs when amniotic fluid enters the circulation, usually via a rent in the amniotic membranes. The features of the syndrome are related both to the mechanical obstruction caused by the components of amniotic fluid and their thromboplastic properties. Amniotic fluid embolism may be associated with coma, convulsions and coagulopathy.

Multiparity is a predisposing factor to this rare condition (1 in 80 000 pregnancies) which usually occurs during labour. Mortality is high (80%) and diagnosis often made at postmortem.

Diagnosis. The features of amniotic fluid embolism include:

- Respiratory distress
- Hypoxia
- Cardiovascular collapse
- Coagulopathy
- Haemorrhage
- Convulsions

- Coma
- Fetal squames seen in the sputum and amniotic fluid in the CVP line aspirate

Management. As part of the treatment of amniotic fluid embolism the patient should be given:

- Cardiorespiratory support: mechanical ventilation; cardiac massage; inotropic support
- Anticonvulsants, diazepam 10–20 mg as required
- Blood to replace blood loss
- Blood component therapy for the management of the coagulopathy as directed by an experienced haematologist

Air embolism. Significant air embolism can occur very rarely during caesarean section. Predisposing factors include Trendelenberg position, hypovolaemia, placenta praevia or abruption. Air embolism causes frothing of blood in the right ventricle making ejection of blood into the pulmonary circulation ineffective.

Diagnosis. Features of an air embolism include:

- Hypotension
- Hypoxia
- Tachypnoea
- Fall in end-tidal carbon dioxide
- Arrhythmias
- Increase in CVP
- 'Mill-wheel' murmur
- Positive findings with pre-cordial Doppler

Management. When air embolism is suspected:

- Put the patient head down in the left wedged position to collect air in the apex of the right ventricle
- Flood the wound
- Aspirate the right atrium via a CVP line if practicable
- Provide cardiorespiratory support as required

Cyanosis

Definition. Cyanosis is a blue discolouration of the skin or mucous membranes. Most observers can detect the sign when the concentration of reduced haemoglobin exceeds 5 g/dl.

Causes. From the oxygen dissociation curve (Figure 3.2) it is evident that the degree of saturation of haemoglobin is a reflection of PaO_2. Cyanosis can be detected by most clinicians in about 95% of patients who have saturations of 89% which corresponds to a PaO_2 of approximately 7.5 kPa. The commonest cause of cyanosis is hypoxaemia although other rare

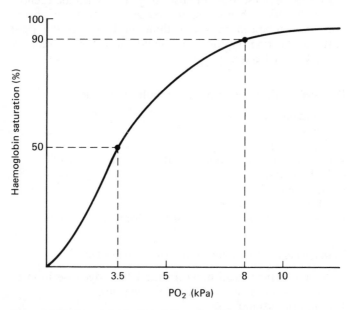

Figure 3.2 Oxyhaemoglobin dissociation curve showing oxygen tensions when the haemoglobin molecule is 50% saturated (P50) and 90% saturated (P90).

causes such as methaemoglobinaemia secondary to prilocaine overdose (>8 mg/kg) should be considered.

Causes of hypoxaemia.
- Reduced haemoglobin saturation due to
  —hypoventilation
  —hypoxic inspired gases
  —ventilation–perfusion mismatch
- Reduced cardiac output as a result of
  —haemorrhage
  —aortocaval compression
  —cardiac failure
- Reduced pulmonary blood flow secondary to
  —pulmonary and other emboli
  —pulmonary hypertension
- Increased oxygen consumption
  —pregnancy
  —malignant hyperthermia

Physiological significance. The observation of cyanosis should suggest hypoxaemia until proved otherwise. Hypoxia if untreated will have deleterious effects on both mother and fetus.

Detection of hypoxia in the anaemic parturient may be difficult because cyanosis will only appear if at least 5 g/dl of reduced haemoglobin is present.

The head down position sometimes required during caesarean section causes venous congestion and cyanosis in the head and neck region which inaccurately reflects the degree of arterial oxygenation.

Pigmented skin and mucous membranes make detection of cyanosis difficult especially in suboptimal lighting such as may occur in some delivery rooms.

Diagnosis. Inspection of the buccal mucosa is the most reliable way of observing cyanosis. The colour of blood in the wound is a useful indicator of saturation of haemoglobin. Adequate saturation of haemoglobin should be confirmed by pulse oximetry or arterial blood gases.

Management. Problems with ventilation are the most frequent causes of hypoxia under general anaesthesia and in the post-operative period. Problems encountered include:

- Oesophageal intubation
- Endobronchial intubation
- Blocked or kinked tracheal tube
- Disconnection of breathing circuit
- Bronchospasm
- Pneumothorax

They should be rapidly excluded and the cause treated:

- Give 100% oxygen (check inspired gas FiO_2)
- Ventilate manually
- Ensure bilateral chest movement
- Confirm appropriate end-tidal carbon dioxide
- Examine both sides of the chest to exclude: bronchospasm, pneumothorax or pulmonary oedema.

If there is no improvement with the lungs being adequately ventilated with 100% oxygen causes of ventilation–perfusion mismatch, e.g. pulmonary embolism (q.v.) should be sought.

Reduced cardiac output should be suspected if associated signs are present: tachycardia, low blood pressure, pallor of membranes.

Haemorrhage (q.v.) is the most likely cause of a reduced cardiac output and should be treated accordingly.

When oxygen supply is marginal the increased oxygen consumption of pregnancy may contribute to hypoxaemia and delivery of the fetus is followed by an improvement in maternal oxygenation.

Convulsions

Definition.   Convulsions or seizures are the clinical manifestations of a paroxysmal excessive discharge of cerebral neurones. They are either generalized or partial and consciousness may or may not be lost during either type.

The most commonly seen type of generalized convulsion is the grand-mal seizure, and is the one we will concentrate on in this section.

Epilepsy is the repeated and continued tendency towards having seizures.

Physiological significance. Convulsions may occur *de novo* in pregnancy in the eclamptic patient or as a presenting symptom of a condition unrelated to pregnancy, e.g. cerebral tumour. More frequently they are seen in the known epileptic for whom pregnancy presents problems which require the coordinated attention of obstetrician, neurologist and sometimes anaesthetist.

Most epileptic women suffer no deterioration of seizure control during pregnancy but a few, particularly those with severe seizure disorders, experience a higher frequency of convulsions.

The pharmacokinetic changes of pregnancy: increased renal excretion, accelerated hepatic metabolism, decreased protein binding and increased volume of distribution tend to cause a decrease in the plasma concentration of anticonvulsant drugs.

Pre-eclampsia, abruptio placenta, induced labour and peripartum haemorrhage are more likely in the epileptic parturient.

During the tonic phase of a generalized convulsion the sustained contraction of muscles markedly increases oxygen consumption while at the same time preventing respiratory movements. The result is the rapid onset of hypoxia, which will occur more quickly in the pregnant patient. This has self-evident implications for both mother and fetus. The associated loss of muscle coordination during a convulsion increases the likelihood of regurgitation of gastric contents and acid aspiration (q.v.).

Diagnosis. Grand-mal seizures are characterized by two distinct phases: initially a sudden loss of consciousness and control of muscle tone and posture in which the body becomes rigid (tonic phase), lasting from a few seconds to a few minutes; followed by the rhythmic contraction of the limb and trunk muscles (clonic phase).

Management. Convulsions occurring in the obstetric patient should be assumed to be eclamptic in origin until proved otherwise. The immediate management of a generalized seizure is the same irrespective of aetiology:

1. Place the patient in wedged position, ideally head down to avoid aspiration and caval compression
2. Clear and maintain the airway
3. Administer 100% oxygen by facemask
4. Stop the convulsion with anticonvulsants
   a. diazepam 0.1–0.2 mg/kg i.v. or p.r.
   then
   b. phenytoin 10–15 mg/kg slowly i.v.
   or
   c. chlormethiazole 0.8% 0.5–1.5 ml/kg i.v.
   if the others are ineffective

If adequate oxygenation cannot be achieved give thiopentone (3–5 mg/kg) i.v., suxamethonium (1–1.5 mg/kg) i.v., intubate (remember to apply cricoid pressure and avoid caval compression) and ventilate.

In *status epilepticus* there is no return of consciousness between convulsions and a great risk of cardiorespiratory decompensation secondary to repeated convulsions or the depressant effects of anticonvulsant therapy. Suitable intensive therapy should be instituted after consultation between senior members of the anaesthetic, obstetric and neurological teams.

Management of labour and delivery. Anaesthetists may be asked to institute extradural analgesia in parturients with known epilepsy during labour. There is no contraindication to the use of local anaesthetics in epileptic patients but special care should be taken because high plasma levels can lower the threshold for convulsions.

When providing general anaesthesia in the epileptic patient or eclamptic patient thiopentone should be the induction agent of choice because of its potent anticonvulsant properties. The depressant effects of recently administered anticonvulsants means the anaesthetist needs to tailor the dose of anaesthetic drugs accordingly to avoid excessive post-operative sedation.

Epileptiform discharges may occur and be masked during anaesthesia so it should be remembered that the post-ictal phase following a seizure during general anaesthesia is a rare cause of delayed recovery from anaesthesia.

Anaphylactoid reactions

Definition. Anaphylactoid reactions are an abnormal multi-system response to the administration of a drug or drugs. The response is not dose related, and as such distinct from a toxic reaction to the drug. The mechanism of the response may or may not be immunological or follow previous exposure to the drug.

Diagnosis. The involvement of several systems in an anaphylactoid reaction causes a multitude of clinical manifestations, some or all of which may be present. In order of frequency, the features of a life-threatening anaphylactoid reaction are:

- Cardiovascular
  —collapse
  —vasodilation
  —dysrhythmias
- Respiratory
  —bronchospasm
  —pulmonary oedema
- Cutaneous:
  —erythema
  —urticaria
  —rash

- Oedema
  - —generalized
  - —supraglottic and laryngeal oedema
- Gastrointestinal
  - —abdominal pain
  - —diarrhoea and vomiting

Physiological significance. The incidence of anaphylactoid reactions is greater in the female population, although it is unclear whether pregnancy has any effect on the incidence, manifestations or outcome of such reactions.

Most cases of anaphylactoid reaction are well tolerated by the patient even without treatment. In a small number of cases severe cardiovascular collapse might lead to cerebral hypoxia and death if untreated.

Such changes in the parturient will have obvious deleterious results on the outcome of any pregnancy including precipitation of premature labour and damage or death of the fetus.

Management. The anaesthetist may be confronted with problems related to anaphylaxis, either being called upon to resuscitate a patient undergoing an anaphylactic reaction, sometimes after exposure to drugs administered during anaesthesia, or when asked to be involved in the obstetric management of a parturient with a past history of anaphylaxis.

The pre-anaesthetic assessment should include direct questioning about a history of allergy, atopy and asthma. Any history of allergic reaction should be examined in detail to elicit any of the features listed above. A convincing history of serious reaction warrants further investigation with cutaneous testing to establish the nature of the drug responsible for a reaction. Such a course of action is time consuming and often in obstetrics such time is unavailable because of the urgent nature of clinical situation. When action is required immediately the anaesthetist should have prepared a course of action which will allow the patient to be managed as safely as is reasonably possible. The following is recommended:

(a) *Avoidance of anaphylaxis*
- Avoid any drugs documented as having caused a reaction
- Regional anaesthesia should be considered, avoiding ester local anaesthetics and those containing metabisulphite as preservative.
- Provide prophylactic regimens: including H_1 (chlorpheniramine 10 mg i.v.) and H_2 receptor antagonists (ranitidine 50 mg i.v.) and hydrocortisone (100 mg i.v.)
- Use etomidate as i.v. induction agent
- Volatile agents are safe
- Muscle relaxants are the drugs most frequently implicated in anaphylactic reactions related to anaesthesia. Suxamethonium is the commonest agent found to cause a reaction but is difficult to avoid in obstetric anaesthesia. Vecuronium or pancuronium are the non-depolarizing muscle relaxants of choice.
- Some opiate analgesics such as omnopon and morphine cause release of histamine and so fentanyl is recommended
- Fluids: use crystalloid rather than colloid solutions where possible to avoid the possibility of reaction to the colloid proteins

(b) *Treatment of an anaphylactoid reaction*
Treatment of an anaphylactic reaction is generally supportive. Intravenous or subcutaneous adrenaline is the drug of choice for the management of both hypotension and bronchospasm. In the event of a suspected anaphylactoid reaction do the following:

1. Summon senior help and warn the intensive therapy unit
2. Assess the need for cardiovascular support by feeling for pulse, measuring BP and look for the extent of any oedema
3. Achieve good venous access (14G or 16G peripheral line) and give i.v. fluids: crystalloid for mild reactions; colloid for more severe cases. More than 2 litres of colloid may be required

4. Give adrenaline 0.1–0.5 mg slowly i.v. or s.c. when hypotension is unresponsive to fluid therapy
5. Insert central venous line for monitoring and drug and fluid administration
6. Monitor ECG and treat arrhythmias as appropriate
7. Consider inotropic support if acute myocardial failure develops

If bronchospasm is present:

1. Assess the severity of any bronchospasm clinically, looking for respiratory distress, tachypnoea, wheeze and cyanosis
2. Give:
   —adrenaline if not already given for cardiovascular support
   —chlorpheniramine 10–20 mg i.v.
   —start aminophylline 6 mg/kg slowly i.v
   —add nebulized salbutamol 2.5–5 mg if required
3. Check arterial blood gases
4. If clinical situation deteriorates perform tracheal intubation following a rapid sequence induction with etomidate (0.15–0.2 mg/kg) and suxamethonium (1–1.5 mg/kg) if not contraindicated and start mechanical ventilation while continuing bronchodilator therapy

Tracheal intubation may be difficult if there is laryngeal oedema and might require a smaller tracheal tube. If impossible perform cricothyroidotomy.

If severe bronchospasm persists further therapies should be considered including:

• Volatile agents such as isoflurane. Do not use halothane if adrenaline has been given because of the risk of dysrhythmias
• Ketamine (50 µg/kg/min)

The anaesthetist should arrange for the patient to have cutaneous testing four to six weeks following a reaction, and where possible radio-immunoassay tests (RAST), leucocyte and basophil histamine release tests. These should provide details about the type of reaction and drugs to which the patient is sensitive. A letter should be given to the patient giving details of the reaction, drugs administered and results of the tests performed. This letter should be updated following subsequent anaesthetics. The patient should be advised to wear a warning bracelet.

Difficult intubation

The complications associated with difficulties of intubation remain the commonest causes of maternal morbidity and mortality associated with general anaesthesia.

Most of the fatalities are related to the inexperience of the anaesthetist involved. Because the incidence of failed intubation is small (1:300) any individual anaesthetist's practical experience of the scenario will be limited. It is vital therefore that the trainee anaesthetist has thought about the possibility and is familiar with a plan of action for the management of a difficult or failed intubation. The essentials of management are maintenance of adequate oxygenation and having a low threshold for abandoning further attempts at intubation, and asking for senior assistance.

Definition. A spectrum of difficulty of intubation exists, from easy through difficult to impossible.

Diagnosis. Ideally the anaesthetist should be able to predict from a history and examination that intubation may be difficult and should be able to plan an appropriate course of action, often with the assistance of a senior colleague.

Several means of assessment at the bedside have been developed as predictors of ease of intubation, including the Malampatti test (see Figure 3.3) and Patil's measurement of

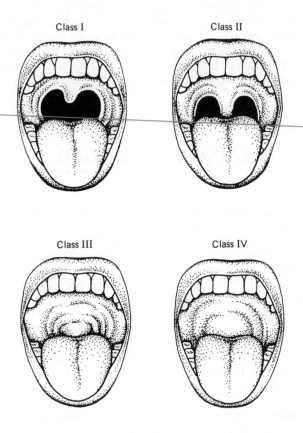

Figure 3.3 Malampatti classification for the prediction of difficult intubation. Assessed after asking patients to open their mouth and protrude their tongue maximally.

Class I: soft palate, fauces, uvula and sillans visible.
Class II: soft palate, fauces and uvula visible.
Class III: soft palate and base of uvula visible.
Class IV: soft palate not visible.

Difficult intubation

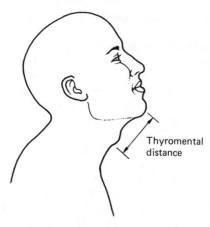

Figure 3.4 Patil's thyromental distance.

thyromental distance (see Figure 3.4). None of these tests have predictive values of 100%, and there is a significant number of false positives but this is an inherent safety feature of the tests. Sometimes diagnosis of difficult intubation is only made when an attempt is made, often following a rapid sequence induction technique.

Significance. As well as risks of aspiration the pregnant woman is more prone to developing hypoxia, due to an increased rate of oxygen consumption and smaller stores of oxygen in a reduced functional residual capacity. She will become hypoxic more quickly when apnoeic during attempts at intubation. This has obvious implications for maternal and fetal well-being.

The parturient is at increased risk of regurgitation and possible aspiration of gastric contents and any delay in securing her airway with a cuffed tracheal tube because of difficulties with intubation will further increase the likelihood of this potentially fatal complication.

General anaesthesia is often performed as an emergency in the obstetric patient because of fetal compromise and a delay in intubation and therefore surgery will increase the risk to the fetus.

Multiple attempts at laryngoscopy and intubation may cause cut lips, broken teeth, lacerations of soft palate and pharynx and oedema of the vocal cords. Some of these may have only cosmetic, though distressing consequences but bleeding and oedema of the upper airway can lead to post-operative respiratory difficulties (q.v.).

Causes. The difficulty of intubation is a reflection of the patient features, the urgency of the situation, the equipment available and the skill and experience of the intubator. The problem for the trainee anaesthetist is that the urgency with which a pregnant mother needs to be intubated may appear to change an easy intubation into a difficult one and a difficult one into an impossible one.

Patient. Features of the patient which may make intubation difficult include:

- Pre-gravid anatomical abnormalities
- A full set of teeth
- Obesity
- Large breasts
- Laryngeal oedema

Intubator. The incidence of difficulty of intubation is related to inexperience of the intubator.

Situation. The circumstances and position which may make intubation of the parturient difficult include:

- Lateral tilt
- Urgent caesarean section
- Incorrect application of cricoid pressure (Figure 3.5)

Management of difficult intubation. The management of a parturient who is expected or proves to be difficult to intubate is set out in an algorithm shown in Figure 3.6.

86

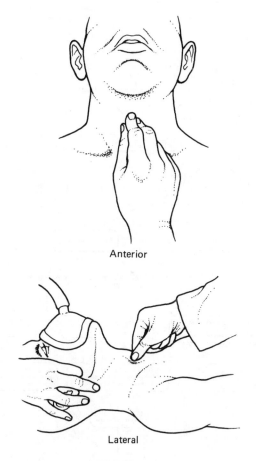

Anterior

Lateral

Figure 3.5 Application of cricoid pressure.

Problems in Obstetric Anaesthesia

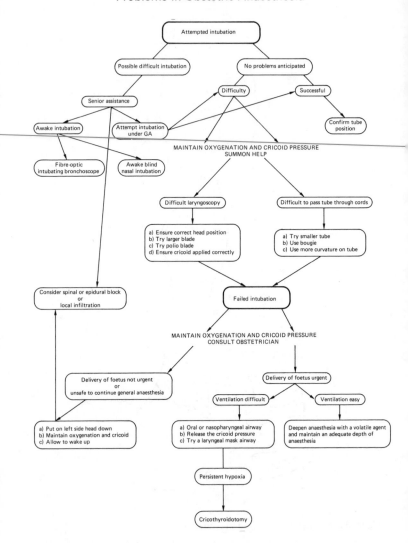

Figure 3.6 An algorithm for the management of difficult and failed intubation.

Confirmation of tracheal tube position is essential because of the risk of inadvertent oesophageal intubation. Various methods are available including:

- Visualization of tube passing through the vocal cords which is often not possible
- Observation of chest movement which may be difficult in the parturient
- Auscultation of breath sounds in both axillae
- End-tidal CO_2 tension
- Oesophageal detector device

Difficulties with intubation may be associated with post operative respiratory difficulties (q.v.) such as stridor.

Aspiration of gastric contents

Aspiration of gastric contents remains a source of maternal morbidity and mortality. The obstetric population are at particular risk of aspiration because of:
- The increased likelihood of regurgitation of gastric contents due to:
  —the urgent nature of the interventions requiring general anaesthesia
  —increased gastric volume due to delayed gastric emptying during labour because of pain and anxiety and opiate administration.
  —raised intragastric pressure
  —incompetent gastro-oesophageal sphincter
- Potential difficulties during intubation

Definition. There is a critical volume (0.3 ml/kg) and pH (<2.5) of gastric contents which if aspirated is likely to result in aspiration pneumonitis.

Diagnosis. Aspiration pneumonitis may be anticipated when aspiration has been witnessed, but may be a retrospective diagnosis as symptoms may develop following silent aspiration.

The clinical picture has a spectrum ranging from rapid onset of cyanosis and circulatory collapse to a more slowly developing picture of respiratory compromise.

Features of the syndrome include:

- Bronchospasm
- Tachypnoea
- Hypoxia with an increased A–a gradient
- Blood stained pulmonary oedema
- Circulatory collapse
- Metabolic acidosis
- Chest X-ray changes
  —fluffy opacities
  —initially affecting dependent areas
  —later becoming generalized

Physiological significance. The respiratory sequelae of aspiration depend on the nature of the fluid entering the lower respiratory tract.

Particulate matter may cause mechanical obstruction of the bronchi and collapse distal to the obstruction. Finer particles may cause shift of fluid into the alveoli often several hours after aspiration. Later (48 hours) these smaller particles can produce an obstructive bronchiolitis due to bronchial oedema.

Acidic fluid entering the bronchi causes degeneration of bronchial epithelium, alveolar necrosis and thrombosis of segmental branches of the pulmonary arteries. The rapid influx of protein rich fluid into the alveolar space can lead to acute hypovolaemia.

The acute response may progress to an adult respiratory distress syndrome picture, and later to permanent parenchymal damage.

Prevention. Prevention of aspiration pneumonitis involves addressing the predisposing factors for regurgitation and aspiration.

Avoidance of general anaesthesia. The use of regional anaesthesia wherever possible avoids the need for intubation and risk of aspiration.

Gastric volume. A critical volume of about 0.3 ml/kg of gastric contents is required to produce pneumonitis.

A controlled dietary regimen during labour, restricting the intake of solid food, will limit any increase in the volume of gastric contents. Where urgent reduction of gastric volume is required, physical and pharmacological methods should be considered:

- Aspiration of gastric contents via a large bore gastric tube
- Metoclopromide i.v. is only effective if given before opiates

Gastric pH. If the pH of the gastric contents can be increased to pH>2.5 the risk of pneumonitis is minimized. Maintenance of gastric pH above this critical level is achieved with regular use of H_2-receptor antagonists (Ranitidine 50 mg i.v. 8 hourly) and non-particulate alkalis (30 ml of 0.3 M sodium citrate orally 4 hourly throughout labour). The use of a single dose of H_2-receptor antagonist just prior to induction of anaesthesia provides protection in the immediate post-operative period when aspiration may also occur.

Lower oesophageal sphincter (LOS). The tone of the LOS can be maintained by the use of i.v. metoclopramide and avoidance of anticholinergic agents.

Anaesthetic technique. The use of a rapid sequence induction prevents vomiting on induction. Effective application of cricoid pressure should preclude passive regurgitation of gastric contents into the pharynx.

Management. Not all patients who aspirate gastric contents develop aspiration pneumonitis but all patients where aspiration is suspected should be monitored clinically for 24 hours, have a chest X-ray immediately after the event and a repeat film if symptoms of aspiration develop.

When aspiration is witnessed or suspected:

1. Clear the airway
   —position the patient head down in the lateral position
   —clear the mouth and pharynx
   —intubate if possible
   —give 100% oxygen
   —suction through the tracheal tube
   —perform bronchoscopy only to remove large particles
2. Maintain gas exchange
   —increase inspired oxygen concentration to keep SaO_2 >94%
   —treat acute bronchospasm with salbutamol (2.5–5 mg nebulized) and aminophylline (6 mg/kg slowly i.v.)
   —use IPPV and PEEP as required
3. Correct acute intravascular fluid losses
4. Give prophylactic antibiotics
   —benzylpenicillin (1.2 g i.v. q.d.s.)
   —gentamicin (80 mg i.v. t.d.s.)
   —metronidazole (500 mg i.v. t.d.s.).
5. Perform a chest X-ray
6. Transfer to intensive therapy unit if further cardio-respiratory support is required

Post-operative respiratory difficulties

Definition.   A variety of respiratory difficulties may occur in the post-operative period including:

- Upper airway obstruction
- Laryngeal obstruction
- Bronchospasm
- Pulmonary oedema

The physiological and pathological changes of pregnancy put the post-operative parturient at particular risk of post-operative respiratory problems.

The facilities for recovery on a labour ward may not be optimal. Mothers may be recovered in an isolated delivery room by a midwife who also has responsibility for the newborn. This makes it vital that the anaesthetist excludes any immediate post-operative respiratory problems and hands over to a person who can effectively monitor the patient in the post-operative period.

Physiological significance. The increased metabolic require-ments of the pregnant woman persist well into the postpartum period. Any respiratory insufficiency of significant duration will impair gas exchange and rapidly lead to hypoxia, hypercarbia, dysrhythmias, eventual cardiac arrest and possible damage to vital organs.

Causes and management of respiratory difficulty. The causes of respiratory difficulties most frequently seen in the immedi-ate post-operative period include:

Upper airway obstruction

Causes:
- The tongue falling against the posterior pharynx
- Collapse of the upper airway soft tissues
- Foreign bodies

The tongue and upper airway soft tissues are the commonest sources of airway obstruction. In the pregnant woman the mucosae of the upper airways are congested particularly in pre-eclamptic and obese women.

Diagnosis:
Features of upper airway obstruction are: lack of air move-

93

ment, snoring, suprasternal and intercostal recession, abdominal movement without chest expansion and cyanosis.

Management:
Several measures should be immediately taken to reverse the airway obstruction including:

- Administration of face-mask oxygen
- Anterior thrust of the mandible
- Putting the patient in the lateral decubitus position
- Insertion of an oro- or nasopharyngeal airway

If these measures do not rapidly improve oxygenation then proceed to tracheal intubation or if impossible perform cricothyroidotomy.

Laryngeal obstruction

Causes:
- Laryngospasm
- Laryngeal oedema
- Foreign body

Laryngeal oedema may be present in the pre-eclamptic mother and may cause difficulties with intubation. Difficulty with intubation may itself result in damage to and oedema of the supraglottic region.

Diagnosis:
Laryngeal obstruction results in stridor, use of accessory muscles of respiration and inadequate air movement.

Management:
Laryngospasm is usually caused by irritation of the vocal cords by secretions, blood, foreign bodies including orophar-

yngeal airway or extubation in a light plane of anaesthesia. After giving face-mask oxygen, any possible irritants should be removed by suction or head-down tilt. Continuous positive pressure oxygen via an airtight mask may allow oxygenation until the spasm subsides.

If the above measures are unsuccessful and hypoxia persists or increases, then a small dose of suxamethonium (10–20 mg) should be given, remembering to apply cricoid pressure to avoid regurgitation and aspiration of gastric contents. The relaxation of the vocal cords will allow positive pressure ventilation to be resumed and continued until the relaxant has worn off and adequate spontaneous ventilation has resumed.

Laryngeal oedema may have been noticed at intubation in the pre-eclamptic patient and may be suspected in those for whom intubation had been difficult or traumatic. Stridor is worse on inspiration and may increase with respiratory effort as extratracheal structures are sucked inward by the negative pressure generated in the trachea during inspiration. Treatment involves:

- Giving humidified face-mask oxygen
- Inhalation of nebulized racemic adrenaline (2.25%), 0.5–1 ml in 2 ml of normal saline every 20 minutes as required then 4 hourly
- Dexamethasone 0.25–0.5 mg/kg i.v., prior to extubation in patients suspected of being at risk of laryngeal oedema. If the above are ineffective re-intubation with a smaller tracheal tube under deep inhalational anaesthesia may be necessary

Bronchospasm

Causes:
- Exacerbation of pre-existing obstructive airways disease
- Aspiration of gastric contents
- Anaphylaxis

Diagnosis:
Bronchospasm is suggested by:

- Respiratory distress
- Tachypnoea
- Hyperexpanded chest
- Expiratory rhonchi

Wheezing in the intubated patient may not be broncho-spastic in origin and other causes should be excluded: obstructed tracheal tube due to clot or mucus, foreign body, overinflated cuff; kinked tube, biting down on tube; congestive cardiac failure; tension pneumothorax.

Management
The aims of management of bronchospasm comprises:

- Maintenance of adequate oxygenation
- Treatment of the underlying precipitant and symptomatic treatment of the bronchospasm depending on the degree of respiratory compromise
- Positive pressure ventilation to support respiration if necessary

Drug therapy includes:

- Nebulized salbutamol, 2.5–5 mg in 2 ml normal saline
- Aminophylline, loading dose 6 mg/kg slowly i.v. over 30 minutes, then 0.5–1 mg/kg/hour as maintenance
- Hydrocortisone, 1–1.5 mg/kg i.v. 8 hourly

Pulmonary oedema.   Pulmonary oedema is an unusual but occasional cause of post-operative compromise.

Causes:
- Pre-eclampsia

    —the hypoproteinaemia of pre-eclampsia may result in non-cardiogenic pulmonary oedema
- Cardiac failure
  —cardiomyopathy of pregnancy
  —pre-eclampsia
  —myocardial infarction
- Fluid overload following treatment of haemorrhage

Diagnosis:
Pulmonary oedema should be suspected when the following features are seen:

- Tachycardia
- Tachypnoea
- Hypoxia and cyanosis despite increasing inspired oxygen concentration
- Wheeze and basal crepitations
- Fluffy shadowing on chest X-ray

Management
The principles of management are correction of hypoxia and treatment of the underlying cause. The patient should be treated in an intensive therapy unit where they can be invasively monitored and receive appropriate cardiovascular and respiratory support.

- Correction of hypoxia
  —high inspired oxygen therapy to maintain $PaO_2 > 8$ kPa
  —continuous positive airway pressure (CPAP) mask
  —positive pressure ventilation with added positive end expiratory pressure (PEEP)
- Diuretic therapy
  —frusemide 0.5–1 mg/kg i.v.
  —dopamine 2–5 µg/kg/min i.v.
- Inotropic and vasodilator therapy
  —dobutamine 10–20 µg/kg/min i.v.
  —glyceryl trinitrate 5–50 µg/kg/min

Resuscitation of the neonate

There are occasions when the anaesthetist is called upon to help in or initiate the resuscitation of a recently delivered neonate.

They may be the only appropriately trained clinician on the labour ward or in theatre who is free to help with resuscitation because both paediatrician and obstetrician are busy elsewhere or the need for resuscitation was unexpected. If a baby requires resuscitation the anaesthetist is primarily responsible for the care of the anaesthetized mother and if she is unstable, attention should be directed to her well-being before that of the neonate. Midwives should be proficient in basic resuscitation techniques.

A teaching programme for all professional personnel working on the labour ward has been produced by a joint working party of members of British Paediatric Association, Royal College of Anaesthetists, Royal College of Obstetricians and Gynaecologists and Royal College of Midwives. This programme describes two levels of resuscitation skills: basic and advanced.

Proficiency in basic resuscitation should ensure the successful management of most emergencies occurring in the newborn.

Advanced resuscitation should only be carried out by those persons skilled in basic resuscitation and who regularly use their skills i.e. paediatricians and anaesthetists.

This section deals with the assessment of the neonate and provides algorithms for basic resuscitation thus allowing the anaesthetist to initiate and assist in the resuscitation of the newborn. For further details the reader is referred to the manuals produced for the training programme described.

Assessment of the neonate. Check that there is:

• Good lung expansion and spontaneous respiratory rate of 40–60/min

- Good oxygenation and that the baby is pink and well perfused
- Normal circulation and easily palpable pulses 120–160/min
- Adequate maintenance of temperature >36°C
- Good tone and spontaneous movement of the baby

If all these are present then resuscitation is not necessary and the baby should be wrapped up in a warm dry blanket and handed to the mother or midwife.

Equipment for basic resuscitation. There should be:

- A resuscitation surface which should be firm, dry, in an ambient temperature of 24–26°C and tilting
- A radiant heat source
- A controllable oxygen source and oxygen funnel
- Equipment for positive pressure ventilation
  —self-inflating bag, e.g. Laerdal or Ambu
  —face masks: 00, 0 or 1 Laerdal
  —oral airway: 000 and 00
  —'Y' piece system as alternative to bag
  —a pressure guage
- Feeding tubes FG 6 and 8 to decompress stomach
- Suction equipment
  —suction device
  —pressure guage
  —catheters FG 6, 8, 10
- Syringes
  —2, 5 and 10 ml
  —21 g and 23 g needles
- Drugs
  —neonatal naloxone 20 μg/ml (10 μg/kg i.v.)
  —vitamin K_1 1 mg ampoule
- Dry warm towels
- Stethoscope

As Figure 3.7 shows, advanced resuscitation techniques may be required when basic resuscitation techniques are unsuccess-

Problems in Obstetric Anaesthesia

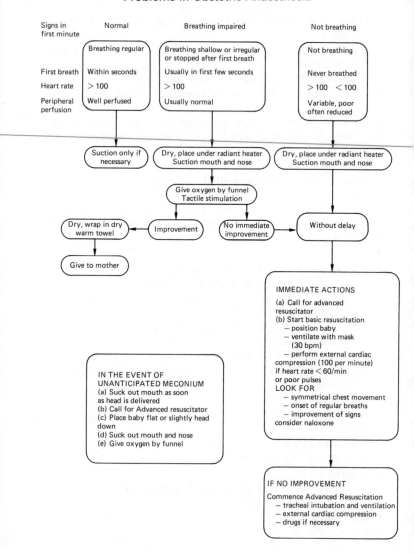

Figure 3.7 Algorithm for the basic resuscitation of the neonate.

ful and their need cannot always be anticipated. There are situations where the presence of personnel with advanced resuscitation skills (e.g. paediatrician) is often needed and should be arranged in advance of delivery. Such situations include:

Abnormalities of labour or delivery
- Fetal distress – suggested by fetal heart rate or acid-base changes and meconium stained liquor
- Caesarean section
- Instrumental delivery
- Abnormal presentation
- Prolapsed cord
- Antepartum haemorrhage
- Prolonged labour

Maternal indications
- Diabetes
- Fever
- Heavy sedation
- Drug dependence
- Coexisting medical condition
- Severe pre-eclampsia

Fetal indications
- Multiple pregnancy
- Preterm labour <37 weeks
- Post-term >42 weeks
- Intrauterine growth retardation
- Isoimmunization
- Abnormal baby

Basic resuscitation may not be adequate to improve the condition of the neonate. In such circumstances other causes for the persistent poor condition of the neonate should be considered in which advanced resuscitation techniques are required, these include:

- Persistent apnoea
- Pneumothorax

- Meconium aspiration
- Diaphragmatic hernia
- Hydrops fetalis
- Blood loss

Advanced resuscitation techniques involve procedures which are not necessary in basic resuscitation and comprise:

- Tracheal intubation
- Positive pressure ventilation
- Decompression of pneumothorax
- External cardiac compression
- Umbilical/peripheral venous cannulation
- Administration of resuscitation drugs
  —sodium bicarbonate 4.2% 5 ml/kg i.v. @ 2 ml/min
  —adrenaline 1:10 000 0.1 ml/kg i.v. or via trachea
  —calcium gluconate 10% 1–2 ml i.v.

It should be emphasized that such procedures should only be performed by experienced personnel.

Miscellaneous

Pre-eclampsia

Pregnancy induced hypertension (PIH), including pre-eclampsia and eclampsia complicates 5–10% of pregnancies. The anaesthetist is frequently called upon to help in the provision of analgesia for labour and vaginal delivery, anaesthesia for caesarean section; the resuscitation of the eclamptic and the intensive care of severe cases of PIH.

Definition.   Pregnancy induced hypertension is diagnosed if two or more of the triad of hypertension, proteinuria and oedema are present, after the 20th week of gestation.

The aetiology of the condition is thought to be an immunological reaction between maternal and fetal tissue at the placental interface.

Physiological significance.   Being a leading cause of maternal mortality and a significant cause of fetal morbidity and mortality PIH poses a serious management challenge to the entire obstetric team.

The involvement of several organ systems makes the manifestations of PIH wide and varied (Table 4.1).

Pregnancy induced hypertension has implications for the fetus including:

- Intrauterine growth retardation
- Prematurity
- Hypoglycaemia
- Intrauterine death

Assessment of PIH.   The following features indicate severe PIH.

History and examination
- Malaise
- Headache
- Epigastric pain and vomiting
- Visual disturbance

Table 4.1 Pathophysiological changes of PIH

Cardiovascular system	Hypertension
	Oedema due to maldistribution of fluid
	Intravascular hypovolaemia
	Increased SVR
	Normal or reduced cardiac output
Respiratory system	Laryngeal oedema
	Pulmonary oedema
Central nervous system	Convulsions
	Cerebral haemorrhage
	Cerebral oedema
Renal system	Proteinuria
	Reduced GFR
	Reduced uric acid excretion
Hepatobiliary system	Abnormal LFTs
	Hypoalbuminaemia
	Hepatic haemorrhage
Clotting system	Thrombocytopenia
	Prolonged thrombin time
	DIC
Placenta	Uteroplacental ischaemia
	Placental abruption

- Diastolic BP >120 mmHg
- Pulmonary oedema
- Twitching/hyperreflexia/clonus
- Papilloedema

Investigations.
- Biochemistry:
  —abnormal urea and electrolytes
  — raised creatinine
  —uric acid >0.4 mmol/l
  —disturbed liver function tests
- Oliguria <0.5 mg/kg/hour
- Proteinuria >3 g/24 h
- FBC and clotting screen
  —thrombocytopenia <100×10^9/l
  —DIC

Management. The treatment of PIH is the termination of the pregnancy and removal of the placenta. The timing of the delivery is based on the risk:benefit ratio to the fetus of the intrauterine and extrauterine environment.

The well-being of the fetus is dependent on the maintenance of adequate placental blood flow.

The mother may be treated with a variety of therapies including:

- Antihypertensives
  Vasodilators
  —methyldopa 250–500 mg p.o. 8 hourly
  —hydralazine 20–40 mg i.v. 4 hourly causes tachycardia
  β-blockers
  —labetalol 5–20 mg i.v. boluses then 0.3–2 mg/kg/hour i.v.i.
  —atenolol 50–100 mg p.o. daily may cause fetal bradycardia and hypoglycaemia
  Calcium antagonists
  —nifedipine 20–40 mg oral/sublingual 8 hourly
- Anti-convulsants
  —diazemuls 10–20 mg i.v. boluses to control fits
  —phenytoin loading dose 10–15 mg/kg i.v.; maintenance
  —100 mg 6–8 hourly
- Sedatives
  —diazemuls 2–10 mg p.o. 8 hourly
  —lorazepam 1–4 mg p.o. 12 hourly
- Aspirin
  low dose aspirin 75–150 mg/24 h may be given to patients with PIH to prevent thrombotic obstruction of the placental blood vessels and improve placental blood flow. It may cause prolonged bleeding times.

Anaesthetic management. The problems for the anaesthetist when managing the analgesic and anaesthetic requirements of the parturient with PIH include:

- Upper airway problems related to oedema
- Hypertensive response to laryngoscopy and intubation

- Interaction of antihypertensive, sedative and anticonvulsant drugs with those used for anaesthesia and analgesia
- Revelation of concealed hypovolaemia by extradural and general anaesthesia
- Associated coagulopathy

Analgesia for labour and vaginal delivery.   In the absence of any contraindication (e.g. coagulopathy) continuous lumbar extradural analgesia is the technique of choice because of improved placental blood flow and attenuation of surges in blood pressure associated with painful contractions. Extradural analgesia is not a hypotensive therapy. The parturient with PIH has a very labile blood pressure and a 500 ml crystalloid preload should be given before institution of block to prevent significant hypotension.

A continuous intravenous infusion of pethidine (10–25 mg/ hour i.v.i.) with Entonox if required is an alternative.

Operative delivery.   Lumbar extradural block with slowly administered increments of local anaesthetic and 1000 ml crystalloid preload is the method of choice.

When regional anaesthesia is inappropriate general anaesthesia is required.

The recommended technique is

1. Pre-oxygenation
2. Cricoid pressure
3. Alfentanil (5 µg/kg) bolus prior to intubation to attenuate the pressor response.
4. Rapid sequence i.v. induction with thiopentone (5 mg/kg) and suxamethonium (1–2 mg/kg)
5. Vecuronium; nitrous oxide/oxygen and isoflurane 0.75–1% inspired concentration
6. If blood pressure control is difficult the use of glyceryl trinitrate as a continuous infusion, 1–5 µg/kg/min (0.3 mg/ kg GTN in 50 ml 5% dextrose at 1–5 ml/h) during the perianaesthetic period is recommended to control hypertension.

Monitoring. In most cases standard monitoring including ECG, non-invasive blood pressure, inspired oxygen concentration, pulse oximetry, end-tidal carbon dioxide tension, and urine output is sufficient. Severe cases in whom fluid management and blood pressure control is difficult require intra-arterial, central venous and possibly pulmonary artery pressure monitoring.

Postpartum. The pathophysiological changes of PIH begin to resolve very soon after delivery of the placenta. Possible postpartum complications the anaesthetist should be aware of are:

- Postextubation stridor due to upper airway oedema – humidified oxygen therapy is usually sufficient
- Re-intubation may be required and difficult
- Continued hypertension
- Convulsions – up to 48 hours postpartum
- Multiorgan failure

All severe cases should be monitored in a high dependency unit during the immediate post-operative period until they are stable, with controlled blood pressure, good urine output and no convulsions. Patients with continuing multisystem failure – pulmonary oedema; renal failure; and coagulopathy require care on an intensive care unit with appropriate invasive monitoring and supportive therapy.

Anaesthesia during pregnancy

Definition. Anaesthesia is required in a small proportion (2%) of pregnant mothers, for both obstetric, such as cervical cerclage and non-obstetric procedures.

Significance. Although infrequent, surgery and anaesthesia during pregnancy has an associated morbidity and mortality for both mother and fetus.

Following laparotomy the incidence of fetal loss is over 20% and after cervical cerclage 30%. For the fetus the risk is inversely proportional to the gestation. In contrast, for the mother the risk of anaesthesia increases with the duration of the pregnancy.

In the first trimester exposure of the fetus to anaesthesia carries the possibility of teratogenesis and termination of the pregnancy. Later in the pregnancy precipitation of premature labour by surgery and anaesthesia presents the greatest danger to the fetus. The aspiration of gastric contents (q.v.) is the major source of morbidity and mortality for the mother after the first trimester.

The greatest threats to fetal well-being during anaesthesia and surgery are, hypoxia, hypotension, hypercarbia, pyrexia, acidosis and electrolyte disturbance.

Management. Elective surgery should be postponed wherever possible. If surgery is required then regional anaesthetic techniques, e.g. spinal anaesthesia for cervical cerclage are preferred to avoid the potential for teratogenicity and acid aspiration pneumonitis.

First trimester
- Mother – providing the mother is not obese and has no history of heartburn then anaesthesia can be performed safely on a face mask if appropriate for the procedure to be performed. Otherwise antacid regimens, rapid sequence induction, cricoid pressure and intubation with cuffed tracheal tube should be part of the anaesthetic technique.
- Fetus – consider carefully the risk:benefit ratio of using agents with known or uncertain teratogenicity: nitrous oxide, H_2-receptor antagonists and metoclopramide. Carefully monitor the mother to avoid conditions harmful to the fetus, e.g. hypoxia, hypotension.

Second and third trimester
- Take measures to prevent acid aspiration (q.v.)
- Avoid aortocaval compression (after 16 weeks for singleton and 12 weeks for multiple pregnancies)
- Treat falls in blood pressure >20% below pre-anaesthetic values.
- Beware instrumentation of congested nasal mucosa, e.g. nasal intubation and nasogastric tubes
- Monitor fetal heart rate as often as is practicable during the peri-operative period

No particular anaesthetic agents have been demonstrated to have advantages over others. The use of thiopentone, suxamethonium, vecuronium, fentanyl and enflurane or isoflurane has the benefit of many years of use without reported ill-effect.

Awareness

The incidence of factual recall during anaesthesia for caesarean section may be as high as 10% using thiopentone, nitrous oxide, oxygen and relaxant, and even with the addition of a volatile agent there remains an incidence of awareness of approximately 1%.

The risk of awareness in the obstetric patient is greater than the general population because of:

- Lack of premedication due to the urgent nature of the operation and fear of neonatal depression
- Use of lower doses of induction and volatile agents to minimize the depression of the neonate and reduction of uterine contractility respectively
- Avoidance of opiate analgesics prior to delivery of the fetus
- Use of high-inspired oxygen concentrations to promote fetal well-being

Definition. The concept of awareness during 'anaesthesia' has extended recently to include not simply factual recall of specified events during anaesthesia and operation but memory of general auditory and painful stimuli. Recall of events may be elicited under hypnosis.

Significance. The most extreme example of awareness is the mother who has complete factual recall of events during her operation and memory of unattenuated pain from the surgical stimulus. The immediate emotional distress caused by such a scenario is obvious. Less clear cut instances of 'awareness' can often not be articulated verbally by the mother and may be manifest as unpleasant dreams and other long-term psychological sequelae such as 'post-traumatic shock syndrome'.

The stress caused by a period of awareness will stimulate the release of large amounts of catecholamines which may cause a reduction in placental blood flow and fetal acidosis.

If reasonable measures have not been taken to prevent awareness then its occurrence may have obvious medicolegal implications for the anaesthetist.

Management

Preparation of mother. As part of the pre-anaesthetic assessment for elective caesarean section under general anaesthesia the small risk of awareness and the reasons for it should be explained to the mother. A similar explanation should be given if time and circumstance allow in the event of an emergency caesarean section. A record of the pre-anaesthetic assessment and discussion should be made in the hospital notes.

Prevention. Prevention of awareness is one of the primary goals of the anaesthetist. The most likely period during which awareness may occur is the time immediately following induction of anaesthesia when plasma levels of induction agent are falling and the alveolar tension of volatile agent is rising. It is important that the anaesthetist's technique during

112

this time is both thorough and rapid. Any delay in intubation and commencement of volatile agent should be covered with additional doses of induction agent.

The use of an inhalational anaesthetic agent is essential to minimize the risk of awareness. The recommended inspired concentration of the different volatile agents are: halothane 0.5%; enflurane 0.6%; and isoflurane 0.75% in a 50:50 nitrous oxide:oxygen mixture. The use of higher inspired concentrations of nitrous oxide and inhalational agent in the first three minutes following induction accelerates the attainment of alveolar concentrations of volatile agent. The use of 50:50 nitrous oxide:oxygen mixtures with recommended inspired concentrations of inhalational agent following this initial period will minimize fetal compromise and uterine relaxation. Following delivery of the fetus the administration of intravenous opiate analgesia and an increase in the inspired concentration of nitrous oxide will reduce the likelihood of awareness during this phase of anaesthesia.

At the end of surgery, to avoid the possibility of the mother waking up paralysed, the volatile agent and nitrous oxide should not be stopped until reversal of neuromuscular block has been achieved and all manipulations including placement of dressings and vaginal toilet have been completed.

Complaints of awareness. In the event of a complaint of awareness it is important to treat any such claims seriously and sympathetically. A full and detailed account should be elicited from the patient and attempts to corroborate the claims should be made from other people present during the events. A consultant anaesthetist should be consulted and involved. If the evidence supports the claim then the clinician involved should explain how and why the awareness may have occurred and should arrange for suitable counselling of the patient. This will often reduce the likelihood of legal action.

Abnormal labour and delivery

Normal labour and delivery is that of a singleton fetus, cephalic presentation, delivered at term, unassisted, via the vagina. The management of abnormal labour and delivery may require the active involvement of the obstetric anaesthetist during labour and at delivery.

Situations include: pre-term labour; multiple gestation, e.g. twins; abnormal presentations, e.g. breech, instrumental delivery, e.g. forceps and cord prolapse. This section deals with some of these circumstances and the implications for parturient, fetus and anaesthetist.

Pre-term labour

Significance. For the *mother* pre-term labour has several implications. The early onset of labour may have been precipitated by potentially harmful conditions such as: intra-uterine or urinary tract infection, placental abruption or intrauterine death. Attempts to arrest premature labour and accelerate the maturation of the fetus with β-receptor agonists and steroids are also potentially harmful to the mother.

Side effects of β-receptor agonists include:

- Tachycardia
- Arrhythmias
- Angina
- Pulmonary oedema
- Hyperglycaemia

Side effects of steroids include:

- Sodium retention
- Hyperglycaemia

The risks to the *fetus* (often multiple) are increased. There is a marked increase in perinatal mortality and morbidity due to respiratory distress, intraventricular haemorrhage and birth trauma.

Management of labour and delivery

Analgesia for labour

Extradural block improves placental blood flow and fetal condition and is therefore the analgesic technique of choice.

Operative delivery

In the absence of excessive tachycardia (>120 bpm, which may limit the capacity of the mother to respond to vasodilation) or any other contraindication lumbar extradural block is advised. Once a decision to deliver the fetus is made all β-receptor agonist therapy should be stopped.

If there is evidence of pulmonary oedema, general anaesthesia with mechanical ventilation and PEEP should be used for delivery, and post-operative transfer to the intensive care unit arranged.

Multiple gestation. The anaesthetist is a vital member of the team responsible for the management of twin, triplet and other multiple deliveries. They should be actively involved early in the labour and be present at the delivery in case anaesthesia is urgently required for instrumental delivery.

When delivering twins, providing both are vertex presentations, vaginal delivery is usually attempted. Where one or more are breech presentation and are estimated to weigh less than 1500 g delivery is by caesarean section. Triplets and greater multiple gestations are all delivered by caesarean section, usually elective unless premature labour occurs.

Physiological significance. For the *mother*, multiple gestations put the mother at increased risk of complications during both antenatal and peripartum periods:

Antenatal period
- Anaemia
- Pre-eclampsia
- Polyhydramnios
- Aortocaval compression
- Placental abruption

- Premature rupture of membranes
- Pre-term labour

Peripartum period
- Hypoxia when supine due to reduced functional residual capacity
- Delayed gastric emptying
- Increased gastric volume
- Instrumental/operative delivery
- Postpartum haemorrhage

The *fetuses* are more likely to be premature; of low birth weight; have a congenital anomaly and the second and subsequent fetus is more likely to suffer birth asphyxia.

Management of labour and delivery. Lateral displacement of the uterus and face-mask oxygen should be maintained throughout labour and delivery and following delivery of the first twin to avoid hypoxia of the the second twin.

When attending multiple deliveries, the anaesthetist should be prepared to provide rapid general anaesthesia to allow urgent delivery or to provide uterine relaxation with a volatile agent.

Analgesia for labour
Lumbar extradural analgesia is the method recommended, avoiding the depressive effects of parenteral opiates on what are frequently immature neonates. It also provides anaesthesia for instrumental delivery if necessary.

Operative delivery
Twins: extradural or subarachnoid block unless contraindicated.
Triplets: careful extradural block or general anaesthesia. Triplets are a relative contraindication to subarachnoid block because of a high incidence of hypotension.

Malpresentation

Definition. This is the presentation at the onset of labour of any part of the fetus other than the vertex. The commonest malpresentation is a breech and is the one dealt with in this section.

Significance. In the later stages of pregnancy subcostal discomfort is greater which may make analgesia difficult to establish.

The fetus is more likely to be premature and there is an increased likelihood of caesarean section.

Management

Analgesia for labour and vaginal delivery
An anaesthetist must be present during attempted vaginal delivery. In the absence of any contraindications, lumbar extradural analgesia is used to provide optimal analgesia throughout the first stage of labour. A top-up for the second stage produces perineal analgesia for episiotomy, allows controlled delivery of the aftercoming head and improves neonatal outcome.

Caesarean section
Extradural or subarachnoid block provide optimal conditions for both mother and fetus. General anaesthesia may be required when regional anaesthesia is contraindicated or refused by the parturient.

Instrumental delivery. Assisted vaginal delivery with either forceps or vacuum extraction (Ventouse) may be indicated when there is:

- Failure to progress
- Malrotation
- Occipitoposterior position

117

- The need to prevent bearing down or limit the maternal work of delivery, e.g. in parturients with pre-eclampsia or cardiorespiratory disease

Management. The aims of anaesthetic management are to provide pain-free contractions, perineal analgesia and pelvic floor relaxation. Attempts should be made to anticipate situations in which instrumental delivery may be required and continuous lumbar extradural analgesia commenced before the second stage of labour.

In the absence of contraindications regional block should be used, aiming to block segments T10 to S5.

Lumbar extradural catheter in situ:
- Check existing level of analgesia and if inadequate:
  —top-up
  —in sitting position
  —give 6–10 ml 2% lignocaine or 0.5% bupivacaine

No extradural catheter in situ
- Single shot subarachnoid block
- Sitting position
- 1.5–2 ml 0.5% heavy bupivacaine

Obstetricians may perform a 'trial of forceps' if they are uncertain of vaginal delivery. This should be performed in theatre and the anaesthetist should be ready to provide suitable anaesthesia for caesarean section, either by extension of an existing block or by general anaesthesia.

Cord Prolapse

Significance. The likelihood of cord prolapse is greater in cases of malpresentation and multiple births. For the fetus cord prolapse poses an immediate threat to life as the umbilical vessels go into spasm and asphyxia ensues.

Management. Cord prolapse is one of the most dramatic obstetric emergencies.

Immediate delivery by caesarean delivery under emergency general anaesthesia is indicated. There is no place for regional anaesthesia.

Examination under anaesthesia.   Placenta praevia is the commonest reason for performing vaginal examination under anaesthesia.

If placenta praevia is suspected and ultrasound assessment of the position of the placenta is inconclusive a vaginal examination is performed by the obstetrician in theatre, if necessary under general anaesthesia, to assess the feasibility of vaginal delivery. If considered feasible amniotomy is performed to induce labour. Where vaginal delivery is considered unsafe, delivery is by caesarean section.

Management.   As there is the potential for torrential haemorrhage during examination, the anaesthetist should be prepared for rapid administration of fluid and induction of anaesthesia for emergency caesarean section. Before examination is performed:

- Give oral antacid therapy 30 ml 0.3 M sodium citrate and H_2 antagonist
- Ensure immediate availability of crossmatched blood
- Transfer to theatre
- Establish venous access via 14G cannula
- Check drugs and equipment for general anaesthesia
- Attach monitoring
  —ECG
  —automated non-invasive blood pressure cuff
  —pulse oximetry
- When ready inform obstetrician that they may start

Because of the risk of severe haemorrhage regional anaesthesia is contraindicated.

Inversion of the uterus.   Inversion of the uterus may occur during the third stage of labour as pressure is applied to the fundus or traction applied to the umbilical cord.

Significance. The danger to the parturient is that of haemorrhage and shock. The condition can be extremely painful as the uterus becomes contracted and engorged. Immediate reduction is imperative to limit such engorgement which may prevent reduction and necessitate hysterectomy.

Management. The aims of initial therapy are resuscitation and include:

- Reassurance and explanation to parturient
- Face mask oxygen 4–6 l/min
- Establishment of fast flowing i.v. infusion of colloid while awaiting arrival of blood
- Urgent crossmatch of at least four units of blood

If replacement of the uterus is impossible under an existing regional block then management should be:

1. Transfer to theatre
2. Administer antacid therapy
3. Application of standard monitoring but including CVP if necessary
4. Careful induction of anaesthesia with etomidate (0.2–0.3 mg/kg) or ketamine (1 mg/kg i.v.)
5. Rapid tracheal intubation applying cricoid pressure

If resuscitation is adequate moderate concentrations of volatile agent may be used to cause uterine relaxation and facilitate reduction of the uterus.

Physiological changes of pregnancy

Appendix 1: Physiological changes of pregnancy

	Direction of change	% change at term	Value at term
Cardiovascular system			
Heart rate	Increased	15	
Systolic blood pressure	Decreased	0–15	
Mean arterial pressure	Decreased	15	
Diastolic blood pressure	Decreased	10–20	
Cardiac output	Increased	40	
Peripheral resistance	Decreased	15	
Blood volume	Increase	35	
Central venous pressure	No change		
Respiratory system			
Tidal volume	Increased	30–40	
Respiratory rate	No change		
Minute volume	Increased	30–40	
Functional residual capacity	Decreased	20	
Oxygen consumption	Increased	20	
Arterial blood gas:			
pH	Increased		7.44
pCO_2	Decreased		4.1 kPa
pO_2	Increased		12.3 kPa
HCO_3^-	Decreased		18–21
Renal system			
Glomerular filtration rate	Increased	25–40	
Renal blood flow	Increased	25–40	
Serum osmolality	Reduced	4–5	
Biochemistry:			
Na	Reduced	4–5	
glucose	Increased	10	
k	No change		
Haematology			
Haemoglobin	Decreased	15	
Haematocrit	Decreased	15	
Platelet count	No change		
White cell count	Increased	10	
Factors:			
II, VII, VIII, IX, X	Increased	Variable	
fibrinogen	Increased	50	
plasminogen activator	Decreased		
antithrombin III	Increased		

Drugs used in obstetric anaesthetic practice

Appendix 2: Drugs used in obstetric anaesthetic practice

Anaesthetic drugs

Thiopentone	3–5 mg/kg
Etomidate	0.2–0.3 mg/kg
Ketamine	1.5–2 mg/kg

Muscle relaxants

Suxamethonium	1.5–2 mg/kg
Atracurium	0.3–0.6 mg/kg
Vecuronium	0.08–0.1 mg/kg

Anticholinesterases

Neostigmine	Reversal treatment of myasthenia (2–3 hours)	i.v. 50 µg/kg i.v. 0.5 mg s.c. 1.5 mg i.m. 0.7 mg p.o. 15 mg
Pyridostigmine	Treatment of myaesthesia (4–6 hours)	Equivalent dose to neostigmine i.v. 2 mg i.m. 3 mg p.o. 60 mg

Opioids

Fentanyl	i.v. 1–5 µg/kg	1–2 hourly
	epidural 50–100 µg	3-4 hourly
Alfentanil	i.v. 5 µg/kg	bolus prior to intubation
Morphine	i.v. 50–100 µg kg	3-4 hourly
	i.m./s.c. 100–200 µg/kg	3-4 hourly
Diamorphine	i.v. 7–10 µg/kg	3-4 hourly
	epidural 5–10 µg/kg	4–6 hourly
Pethidine	i.v./i.m. 0.5–1.5 mg/kg	2–3 hourly
Naloxone	i.v./i.m./s.c. 10–30 µg/kg	20–30 minutes

Appendix 2: Drugs used in obstetric anaesthetic practice

Anti-convulsants

Diazemuls	i.v./p.r. 10–20 mg	
Phenytoin	loading dose i.v. 10–15 mg/kg	daily
	maintenance i.v. 1.5–2 mg/kg	
	p.o. 3–6 mg/kg	
Chlormethiazole	loading dose i.v. 5–10 mg/kg	40–100 ml 0.8% solution
	maintenance i.v. as required	1–4 ml/min

Bronchodilators

Salbutamol	nebulized 2.5–5 mg	4 hourly
	i.v. 0.5 µg/kg/minute	
Terbutaline	nebulized 2–5 mg	
Aminophylline	loading dose i.v. 6 mg/kg	
	maintenance i.v. 0.5–0.7 mg/kg/hr	
Hydrocortisone	i.v. 1.5–5 mg/kg	8 hourly
Prednisolone	p.o. 5–60 mg	daily

Antacid therapy

0.3 M sodium citrate	0.3 ml/kg	4 hourly
Ranitidine	i.v./i.m. 50 mg	8 hourly
	p.o. 150 mg	12 hourly
Cimetidine	i.v. 200–400 mg slowly	6 hourly
	p.o. 200–400 mg	6 hourly

Cardioactive drugs

Adrenaline	i.v. bolus 1 mg ($\equiv$10 ml of 1:10 000)	0.03 mg in 50 ml 5% dextrose
	i.v. 0.01–0.1 µg/kg/min	ml/hr=0.01 µg/kg/min
Atropine	i.v. 2 mg	
Atenolol	i.v. 2.5–10 mg slowly	
	p.o. 50–100 mg daily	

Appendix 2: Drugs used in obstetric anaesthetic practice

Bretylium	loading dose i.v. 5–10 mg/kg maintenance i.v. 1–2 mg/kg	
Calcium chloride 10%	i.v. 10 mls	
Dopamine	i.v. 2.5–5 µg/kg/min	3 mg/kg in 50 mls 5% dextrose ml/hr=µg/kg/min
Dobutamine	i.v. 5–20 µg/kg/min	
Ephedrine	i.v. 10–15 mg i.m. 10–15 mg	
Esmolol	loading dose 1 mg/kg maintenance 50–300 µg/kg/min	5 g in 500 ml 5% dextrose = 10 mg/ml
Glyceryl trinitrate	i.v. 1–5 µg/kg/min	3 mg/kg in 50 mls 5% dextrose ml/hr=µg/kg/min
Hydralazine	i.v. 20–40 mg 4 hourly	
Labetalol	bolus dose i.v. 5–20 mg maintenance i.v. 20-150 mg/hr	0.5% solution= 5 mg/ml
Lignocaine	loading dose i.v. 1 mg/kg maintenance i.v. 1–4 mg/hr	
Methyldopa	p.o. 250–500 mg 8 hourly	
Sodium bicarbonate	50 mls 8.4% (1 mmol/ml) solution dose/mmol=base deficit (mEq/l × wt (kg)/3	following cardiac arrest correction of metabolic acidosis

Appendix 2: Drugs used in obstetric anaesthetic practice

Local anaesthetics

Lignocaine 2% plain	*extradural block:*	
	caesarean section	20–30 ml
	forceps delivery	10–15 ml sitting
Bupivacaine 0.5% plain	*extradural block:*	
	caesarean section	20–30 ml
	forceps delivery	10–15 ml sitting
Bupivacaine 0.25% plain	*intermittent extradural analgesia:*	8–15 ml
	first dose	6–10 ml
	top-up	
Bupivacaine 0.125% plain	*continuous extradural analgesia*	10–15 ml/hour
Bupivacaine 0.5% heavy	*spinal block:*	
	caesarean section	2.5–3.0 ml
	forceps delivery	2.0–2.5 ml sitting

Oxytocics

Prostin E2	induction of labour	3 mg pessary p.v. or 0.25–0.5 µg/min i.v
	termination of pregnancy	2.5–5 µg/min i.v.
Oxytocin	induction of labour	2–12 mUnit/min i.v.
	third stage of labour and postpartum stimulation of the uterus	10–20 u i.v. bolus then 20–100 u in 500 ml 5% dextros at 1–3 ml/min
Syntometrine	third stage of labour	0.5–1 ml i.m./i.v. 1 ml ≈ 5 u oxytoci +0.5 mg ergometrine

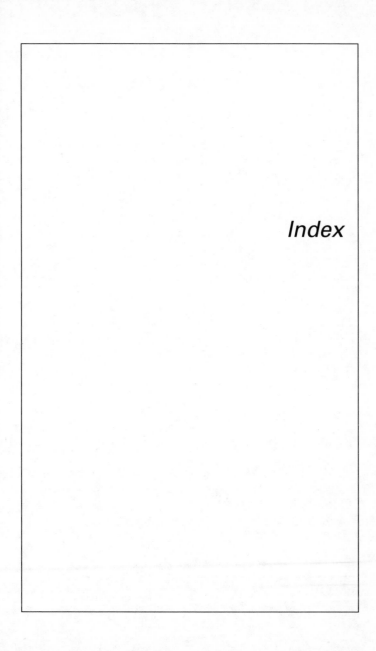

Index

Index

Abnormal presentation, 100, 114
Abnormal uterine anatomy, 61
Abruptio placenta, 60, 77
Acid aspiration, 31, 34, 55, 77, 89
Acidosis, 20, 33, 42, 44, 48, 56, 59, 90, 110, 112
Activated partial thromboplastin time, 66
Adrenaline, 44, 81, 82, 102, 130
Adult respiratory distress syndrome, 90
Advanced life support, 57
Advanced resuscitation of neonate, 98
Air embolism, 71, 73
Airway assessment, 21
Airway difficulties, 26
Airway management, 34
Alfentanil, 7, 108, 129
Aminophylline, 10, 82, 92, 96, 130
Amniotic fluid embolism, 71, 72
Ampicillin, 6, 11
Anaemia, 23, 24, 26, 60, 116
Anaphylactoid reactions, 56, 79, 81, 95
Angina, 114
Antacid therapy, 23, 119
Antepartum haemorrhage, 59, 61, 100
Anti-coagulation, 32
Anti-convulsants, 107
Antibiotics, 6, 11, 51
Anticholinesterase therapy, 15, 16
Anticoagulation, 6, 72
Antihypertensives, 17, 107
Aortic valve disease, 3, 56
Aortic valve insufficiency, 3
Aortic valve stenosis, 3
Aorto-caval compression, 22, 39, 56, 75, 78, 111, 116
Apnoea, 42, 102
Arachnoiditis, 50
Arrhythmias, 3, 4, 7, 42, 73, 114
Arterial blood gases, 10, 11

Aspiration pneumonitis, 43, 89, 90, 91, 110
Aspirin, 65, 107
Asthma, 8
Asystole, 55
Atenolol, 107, 130
Atracurium, 129
Atrial septal defect, 3
Autonomic disturbance, 14
Avascular necrosis, 26
Awareness, 31, 34, 111, 112

Backache, 33, 50
Bacterial endocarditis, 6
Basic life support, 57
Basic resuscitation, 98
Beta-blockade, 7
Birth asphyxia, 116
Birth trauma, 17, 61, 115
Bleeding diathesis, 32
Bleeding time, 66
Blood component therapy, 73
Blood glucose, 18
Blood loss, 21, 22, 34, 62, 102
Blood patch, 47
Blood transfusion, 24, 60
Bloody tap, 40
Bradycardia, 14, 32, 38, 42
Brain damage, 56
Breast feeding, 34
Breech, 32, 114, 117
Bretylium, 44, 131
Broken extradural catheter, 49
Bronchopneumonia, 10, 11
Bronchospasm, 8, 11, 76, 79, 82, 90, 92, 95, 96
Bruising, 66
Bulbar weakness, 15
Bupivacaine, 42, 43, 44, 132

Caesarean section, 17, 18, 21, 24, 31, 36, 57, 100, 105, 111, 115, 117, 119
Calcium chloride, 131
Calcium gluconate, 102
Cardiac arrest, 39, 42, 44, 55, 56, 57, 93

Index

Cardiac failure, 5, 13, 71, 75, 82, 96, 97
Cardiorespiratory disease, 32, 118
Cardiomyopathy, 56, 97
Cardiopulmonary resuscitation, 39, 44, 57
Cardiovascular collapse, 44, 72, 79
Cardiovascular disease, 3, 17
Cardiovascular toxicity, 42
Cauda equina, 51
Central nervous system toxicity, 42
Cerebral haemorrhage, 106
Cerebral oedema, 106
Cerebral tumour, 12
Cerebrovascular disease, 16, 20, 32
Cervical cerclage, 31, 109
Chlormethiazole, 78, 130
Chlorpheniramine, 82
Cimetidine, 130
Clotting factors, 65
Coagulopathy, 49, 60, 61, 72, 108, 109
Coarctation of the aorta, 4
Coma, 72
Complications of diabetes, 17
Complications of immobility, 13
Concealed haemorrhage, 60
Congenital heart disease, 3
Congenital malformations, 6, 17
Contractures, 13
Convulsions, 42, 43, 72, 76, 77, 78, 106, 109
Cord prolapse, 114, 118
Coronary artery disease, 3, 16
CPAP, 97
Cranial nerve palsy, 46
Cricoid pressure, 39, 43, 57, 78, 86, 87, 91, 108, 121
Cricothyroidotomy, 94
Cyanosis, 55, 74, 75, 82, 94, 97

Damage to the bladder, 45
Deep vein thrombosis, 20

Dehydration, 26, 27
Delayed gastric emptying, 22
Dexamethasone, 95
Diabetes, 16, 20, 32, 100
Diamorphine, 129
Diaphragmatic hernia, 102
Diazepam, 43, 78, 107, 130
DIC, 65, 106
Difficult airway, 22
Difficult intubation, 23, 32, 55, 83, 86, 94
Dobutamine, 44, 98, 131
Dopamine, 97, 131
Drowsiness, 42
Drug dependence, 100
Dural puncture, 35
Dural puncture headache, 35, 46, 47
Dyspnoea, 4, 8, 9, 10
Dysrhythmias, 13, 79, 82, 93

Ecchymoses, 66
Echocardiography, 5, 13
Eclampsia, 105
Eisenmenger's syndrome, 3
Embolism, 67
Endobronchial intubation, 76
Entonox, 7, 11, 27, 36, 108
Ephedrine, 39, 44, 131
Epigastric pain, 105
Epilepsy, 77
Erythromycin, 11
Esmolol, 7, 131
Etomidate, 12, 129
Examination under anaesthesia, 119
Exhaustion, 4, 9
Extensive block, 38, 40
Extradural abscess, 51, 52
Extradural analgesia, 6, 11, 19, 22, 27, 31, 33, 35, 78, 108, 116
Extradural block, 7, 14, 19, 31, 33, 45, 48, 49, 51, 108, 115, 117
Extradural catheter, 7, 15, 23, 33, 38, 40
Extradural fentanyl, 48

Index

Extradural haematoma, 40, 49, 51, 67
Extradural opiates, 12
Extradural vein puncture, 40

Failed intubation, 83, 88
Failure of extradural block, 36
Fasting blood glucose, 18
Fentanyl, 129
Fetal asphyxia, 17
Fetal distress, 21, 100
Fetal squames, 72
Fibrin degradation products, 66
Fibrinogen, 66
First trimester, 110
First stage of labour, 31
Foot drop, 50
Forceps delivery, 31, 34, 114
Frusemide, 97

Gag reflex, 13
Gentamicin, 6, 15, 92
Gestational diabetes, 20
Glucocorticoids, 11, 19
Glycaemic therapy, 17, 18, 19
Glyceryl trinitrate, 98, 108, 131
Glycosylated haemoglobin, 18

Haemarthroses, 66
Haematoma, 61
Haemoglobin electrophoresis, 27
Haemoglobinopathies, 25
Haemophilia A, 65
Haemorrhage, 59, 72, 75, 76, 97, 119, 120
Haemostatic failure, 64
Halothane, 12
Headache, 34, 105
Heavy sedation, 100
Henoch-Schönlein Purpura, 65
Heparin, 65, 72
Hepatic haemorrhage, 106
High spinal block, 38, 39
Humidified oxygen, 10
Hydralazine, 107, 131
Hydrocortisone, 11, 96, 130
Hydrops fetalis, 102

Hypercarbia, 93, 110
Hyperglycaemia, 17, 18, 114
Hyperreflexia, 106
Hypertension, 14, 17, 20, 105, 106, 108
Hypoacusis, 46
Hypoalbuminaemia, 106
Hypoglycaemia, 17, 105
Hypotension, 27, 28, 32, 33, 34, 38, 39, 40, 42, 44, 56, 59, 71, 73, 79, 108, 110, 117
Hypothermia, 28
Hypotonic bladder, 45
Hypoventilation, 75
Hypovolaemia, 6, 32, 34, 56, 62, 90, 106, 108
Hypoxia, 17, 20, 25, 27, 42, 56, 59, 71, 72, 73, 74, 75, 76, 85, 90, 93, 97, 110, 116
Hypoxic brain damage, 42

Ideal body weight, 20
Idiopathic thrombocytopenic purpura, 65
Inadequate extradural analgesia, 35, 36
Infection, 27
Inotropes, 44
Instrumental delivery, 32, 50, 100, 114, 115, 116, 118
Insulin, 16, 17, 19
Intrauterine growth retardation, 100, 105
Intrauterine death, 17, 105
Intrauterine death, 114
Intravenous injection of local anaesthetic, 40
Inversion of the uterus, 119
Iron overload, 25

Ketamine, 12, 129
Ketoacidosis, 17
Ketonuria, 18

Labetalol, 107, 131
Laryngeal obstruction, 92, 94

Index

Laryngeal oedema, 80, 86, 94, 95, 106
Laryngospasm, 94
Left-to-right shunts, 3
Lignocaine, 7, 43, 131, 132
Litigation, 36, 112, 113
Liver disease, 20
Loss of consciousness, 38

Malampatti test, 83
Malignant hyperthermia, 75
Malpresentation, 117
Malrotation, 118
Mass motor reflex, 14
Massive extradural injection, 38
Maximum doses of local anaesthetics, 43
Mechanical ventilation, 11, 12
Meconium, 100, 102
Methaemoglobinaemia, 75
Methyldopa, 107, 131
Metoclopramide, 91, 110
Metronidazole, 92
Missed segment, 36
Mixed valve lesions, 3
Morbid obesity, 20
Morphine, 129
Motor block, 32, 35, 38, 40
Multi-organ failure, 109
Multiple gestation, 32, 61, 100, 114, 115
Multiple sclerosis, 13, 14
Muscle twitching, 42
Myasthenia gravis, 15
Myocardial depression, 56
Myocardial ischaemia, 56, 97
Myocardial toxicity, 42
Myotonic dystrophy, 13

Naloxone, 100, 129
Nasal intubation, 111
Nausea and vomiting, 33, 46
Nebulized adrenaline, 95
Neck stiffness, 46
Neonatal hypoglycaemia, 18
Neostigmine, 15, 129
Nephropathy, 16

Neurological deficit, 34, 45, 49
Neurological disease, 12
Neuropathy, 16, 17, 18
Nifedipine, 107
Non-invasive cardiac investigations, 5
Numbness of tongue and mouth, 42
NYHA functional classification of cardiac disease, 5

Obesity, 20, 55, 86, 93
Obstructive airways disease, 95
Occipitoposterior position, 118
Oedema, 4, 5, 80, 90, 105, 108
Oesophageal intubation, 76, 86
Oesophageal reflux, 22
Opiates, 7, 27, 116, 129
Oral hypoglycaemic drugs, 16, 17, 18
Osteomyelitis, 26
Overdose of local anaesthetic, 38
'Oxygen flux', 24, 25
Oxygen therapy, 23, 28
Oxytocin, 132

Pain, 32, 36
Palpitations, 4, 6
Papilloedema, 106
Paraesthesia, 50
Paraplegia, 12, 13, 50
Patent ductus arteriosus, 3, 4
PEEP, 97, 115
Pencil point needle, 46
Perinatal mortality, 26
Perinatal mortality rate, 21
Peripartum cardiomyopathy, 3
Peripartum haemorrhage, 67
Peripheral nerve palsy, 50
Pethidine, 11, 12, 108, 129
Phenytoin, 78, 107, 130
Photophobia, 46
Placenta praevia, 60, 73, 119
Placental abruption, 73, 106, 116
Placental blood flow, 33

Index

Platelet count, 66
Peak expiratory flow rate, 10
Platelet function, 65
Pneumothorax, 10, 76, 96, 102
Polyhydramnios, 116
Post-operative analgesia, 12, 15, 16, 23, 28
Post-operative analgesia, 23, 34
Postpartum haemorrhage, 116
Post-traumatic shock syndrome, 112
Postpartum haemorrhage, 59
Pre-eclampsia, 20, 26, 32, 65, 77, 97, 100, 105, 116, 118
Pre-eclampsia, 56
Pre-eclamptic, 93
Pre-existing cardiac problems, 5
Pre-oxygenation, 23
Pre-term labour, 100, 114, 115, 116
Prednisolone, 130
Pregnancy induced hypertension, 17, 105
Pregnant diabetic, 17
Premature fetus, 32
Premature labour, 80
Premature rupture of membranes, 116
Prematurity, 17, 26, 105
Pressor response to intubation, 7
Pressure areas, 13
Pressure sores, 13
Prolapsed cord, 100
Prolonged labour, 32, 61, 100
Prolonged thrombin time, 106
Prophylactic antibiotics, 28, 92
Propranolol, 15
Prostaglandins, 11
Prosthetic heart valves, 3, 6
Prostin E2, 132
Proteinuria, 105, 106
Prothrombin time, 66
Pulmonary embolism, 20, 56, 71, 76
Pulmonary hypertension, 3, 71, 75

Pulmonary oedema, 6, 76, 79, 90, 92, 96, 97, 106, 109, 114, 115
Pulse oximetry, 75
Pulsus paradoxus, 9, 10
Pyrexia, 9, 14, 100, 110
Pyridostigmine, 129

Ranitidine, 91, 130
Rectal pain, 36
Reduction of the uterus, 121
Reflux, 110
Removal of retained placenta, 31
Renal disease, 17
Renal failure, 25, 109
Respiratory alkalosis, 11
Respiratory depression, 15, 33
Respiratory difficulties, 92, 93
Respiratory failure, 38, 39, 40
Resuscitation, 55, 64, 120
Resuscitation of neonate, 101
Retained products of conception, 61
Retinopathy, 16, 17
Retroverted uterus, 45
Revealed haemorrhage, 60
Right-to-left shunts, 3
Ruptured utero-ovarian vein, 60

Sacral pain, 36
Salbutamol, 10, 82, 92, 96, 130
Second stage of labour, 31, 34
Second trimester, 111
Seizures, 41
Septal defects, 4
Shivering, 35, 48
Shock, 120
Shoulder dystocia, 21
Sickle cell crisis, 25
Sickle cell disease, 25
Sickle cell trait, 25, 27
Slurred speech, 42
Sodium bicarbonate, 102, 131
Sodium citrate, 91, 119, 130
Spinal cord compression, 49
Spinal deformity, 32

Index

Spinal needle, 46
Spinal nerve neuropathy, 50
Spirometry, 10
Status epilepticus, 78
'Stiff joint syndrome', 18, 20
Stridor, 89, 95, 109
Stridor, 94
Subdural block, 40
Subdural haematoma, 47
Streptokinase, 72
Subarachnoid block, 7, 14, 19, 117
Subarachnoid blocks, 31
Subarachnoid catheters, 32
Sudden death, 20
Suprapubic pain, 36, 45
Sweating, 14
Sympathetic block, 32, 36
Syncope, 4, 6
Syntocinon, 11
Syntometrine, 132
Systemic lupus erythematosus, 65
Systemic toxicity, 41, 42

Tachycardia, 5, 71, 76, 97, 114, 115
Tachypnoea, 5, 71, 73, 82, 90, 96, 97
Teratogenesis, 110
Terbutaline, 15, 130
'Test dose', 40
Tetralogy of Fallot, 3, 4
Thalassaemia, 25
Thiopentone, 23, 43, 78, 108, 129
Third stage of labour, 120
Third trimester, 111
Thrombo-embolism, 22
Thrombocytopenia, 65, 67, 106
Thrombolysis, 72
Thrombopathia, 65
Thrombosis, 26
Thrombotic thrombocytopenic purpura, 65
Thyromental distance, 83, 85
Tinnitus, 42, 46
Top-up, 117, 118
Thromboembolism, 20

Total spinal block, 39
Toxic reaction, 35, 43
Tracheal intubation, 7, 31, 43, 55, 82, 102
Transfusion, 24, 27
Trial of forceps, 118
Trial of labour, 32
Triple rhythm, 5
Triplets, 115, 117
Twins, 117

Unconsciousness, 42
Upper airway obstruction, 67, 92, 93
Upper airway reflexes, 13
Urinalysis, 18
Urinary retention, 34, 45
Urticaria, 79
Uterine atony, 61
Uterine contraction, 40
Uterine dysfunction, 32
Uterine inversion, 61
Uterine rupture, 60
Utero-ovarian vein rupture, 61

Vacuum extraction, 118
Valvular lesions, 3
Vancomycin, 6
Vasa praevia, 60
Vasoconstrictors, 6,44
Vasodilation, 32, 36, 56, 79
Vecuronium, 12, 129
Ventilation–perfusion mismatch, 76
Ventilatory support, 8
Ventricular fibrillation, 42, 44, 55
Ventricular septal defect, 3
Ventricular tachycardia, 55
Visual disturbance, 42, 105
Vital capacity, 6, 13, 16
Vitamin K, 100
Vomiting, 105
Von Willebrand's disease, 65

Warfarin, 72
Weight gain, 4
Wheeze, 9